D0095140

Tornado of Life

Tornado of Life: A Doctor's Journey through Constraints and Creativity in the ER

Jay Baruch

The MIT Press

Cambridge, Massachusetts | London, England

The MIT Press would like to thank the anonymous peer reviewers who provided comments on drafts of this book. The generous work of academic experts is essential for establishing the authority and quality of our publications. We acknowledge with gratitude the contributions of these otherwise uncredited readers.

The essays in this book are based in real events but changes have been made to protect patient privacy and confidentiality. These essays should not be taken as giving medical advice.

This book was set in ITC Stone Serif Std and ITC Stone Sans Std by New Best-set Typesetters Ltd. Printed and bound in the United States of America.

Library of Congress Cataloging-in-Publication Data

Names: Baruch, Jay, author.
Title: Tornado of life : a doctor's journey through constraints and creativity in the ER / Jay Baruch.
Description: Cambridge, Massachusetts : The MIT Press, 2022. | Includes bibliographical references and index.
Identifiers: LCCN 2021038778 | ISBN 9780262046978 (hardcover)
Subjects: MESH: Emergencies—psychology | Physician–Patient Relations | Emergency Treatment | Emergency Service, Hospital
Classification: LCC RA975.5.E5 | NLM WB 105 | DDC 362.18—dc23
LC record available at https://lccn.loc.gov/2021038778

10 9 8 7 6 5 4 3 2 1

For Jen and Daniel

We can learn a lot about a person in the very moment that language fails them.

—Anna Deavere Smith, *Talk to Me*

Contents

Part III: Possibility

1
Chief Complaint

"What's bothering you, sir?" I ask Mr. A again. He's like a gentle child, sitting there on the stretcher wearing PJs of Christmas colors. Only he also has a shock of white hair and advanced dementia. I'm unable to find the paperwork from the nursing home that sent him to the ER in the middle of the night. He looks as mystified as I feel.

"Do you know why the nursing home sent you in, sir?"

He answers with bemused eyes and a mischievous smile. I read his chief complaint the triage nurse recorded in his chart one more time—"I feel great."

2
Not the Beginning

My original plan was for you to step into this book without my forecasting what's to come. The ER invites unpredictability. The practice of emergency medicine is a dance with the unexpected. I wanted to simulate that instability, the shaky ground on which we care for patient after patient, broken bodies and broken stories. Defibrillating a lifeless heart is a gripping moment familiar to most television viewers, but it's arguably an easier task than what I believe is a more critical activity, one charged with more dramatic energy: finding the heart of a patient's story and responding to it.

Thinking with stories uses different muscles than thinking about stories. When COVID-19 became the story of medicine and our communities, the unexpected swept into all our lives. For too many, the disruption was overwhelming and irreparable. As a result, we became untethered from the stories that once grounded our lives. In her book *A Paradise Built in Hell*, Rebecca Solnit writes, "The word emergency comes from emerge, to rise out of. . . . An emergency is a separation from the familiar, a sudden emergence into a new atmosphere, one that often demands we ourselves rise to the occasion."

In the ER, where the sliding doors open to innumerable problems, I've lost count of how often I've craved to rise to the occasion only to discover I'm at a loss as to what that means and entails. Finding clarity in those moments resembles the disorientation one feels staring out an airplane window above a bank of clouds and trying to determine the location of the land below. Even though the landscape is inaccessible to the eyes, you're reassured the outlines will come into focus once you dip lower in the sky. Likewise, in my work in the ER, discovering how to rise to the occasion often requires a paradoxical movement of descent.

I was well trained to recognize and treat acutely ill and injured patients. Unfortunately, my patients' bodies didn't always read the same textbooks and journal articles that I did. Their symptoms didn't necessarily point to a disease. Sometimes, patients emptied a trunkload of problems at my feet. Or they were close-lipped and withholding. My training didn't address what turned out to be the most frustrating parts of my emergency medicine practice—working with uncertainty and stories that felt less like nuts to be cracked and more like messy first drafts.

At times, emergency medicine seems like an emotional and moral contact sport. This book represents my efforts to dig into experiences that left me feeling lost or inadequate, confused or ashamed, unsettled or just plain silly. Often, these dilemmas couldn't be resolved without creating another problem. When faced with uncertainty and ambiguity, physicians are inclined to reach for abstract ideas or point to reams of evidence in the medical literature in search of an answer. What a strange instinct, I've always thought: to look for solutions to confusing situations by flying higher and farther away instead of making the necessary movement of descent, asking better questions, and thinking more like a writer.

My work as an emergency physician has always struck me as a fundamentally creative act. Caring for patients demands creativity as a clinical skill. This insight is neither groundbreaking nor original. The medical encounter has been compared to improvisation: it's unscripted and unpredictable, and requires thinking on our feet, curiosity, and following possible threads rather than closing them off.

An ER visit is a significant narrative event in any patient's life, and patients need clinicians who are at least willing and able to engage in that type of recognition. But the ER can be a narrative disaster zone. Communication is hard in crowded spaces, where patients share sensitive information in hallways or within earshot of other patients to physicians and nurses they're meeting for the first time. Moreover, these strangers might be called away unexpectedly by other urgent matters.

Years ago, after I gave a talk at another medical school, an esteemed professor of medicine said, "You're an ER doc. You don't have time for story." He was right. The ER encounter is one where a "pressured listener" tries to understand a "pressured storyteller" while under ever-shifting conditions and constraints. But that doesn't stop people from coming to the ER. And these problems are no longer particular to the ER. Providers in other medical fields and across healthcare wrestle with less time with more patients while staring glassy eyed at computer screens. These obstacles serve as arguments, I explained to the professor, for why creative skills are necessary now more than ever.

Our brains are hardwired for story, and if we're not careful, the story we create may be very different from the one a patient is telling. To be an emergency physician—any clinician, really—is to be a professional listener of stories, which is difficult without insight into how stories work. Medical students spend a semester dissecting the human body, yet they're unaware of the anatomy of stories. And there are only three principal elements to memorize: character, desire, and conflict. Patients are characters in their own stories, motivated by desires and needs, but obstacles get in the way. In the ER, the burdens of the body are amplified and complicated by social, economic, and mental health troubles that are often the source of a person's distress, only they're hidden or buried. These external obstacles are often linked with internal hurdles such as fear, insecurity, even love. The patient in the ugly, uncomfortable gown is a person who, like all of us, is scuffling through inner and outer journeys. When tasked with a cloud of problems, clinicians need creative imagination. We must pivot from "What's wrong with the body" or "What's the answer to this problem" to different questions, namely: "What are the obstacles and the stakes in this person's story and why? How does what happened square with what they expected to happen?" One can't care for patients without working the fields of their expectation gaps.

Stories aren't completed, polished objects given to us. Stories are constructions. Writing reminds me of how hard it can be to put an experience into words. Writing is rewriting for me. Imagine being a patient in a busy ER, sharing personal information with a stranger, finding just the right words when sick, in pain, and possibly terrified of what it all means. A patient's story is often a set of fragments, or a first draft, a best effort in trying circumstances. By telling a story, a patient isn't only describing what happened; they're descending into an experience and trying to understand it. At the heart of emergency medicine, and medicine as a whole, are small stories that are anything but little to the person experiencing them.

The beginning of any story is a platform built for leaping into uncertainty, and this beginning is no different. In this book, I want to bring you inside some experiences that have stood out over my career. The stories don't line up into a neat path. That would be antithetical to what this book is about. Besides, the tension between seemingly misfit pieces is a fertile place for examining the self and the body and the social systems in which they belong. The ability to work with stories is, and will continue to be, the most cost-effective and critical navigation instrument in medical care. The best technology is of little use if we get the story wrong.

I
Vulnerability

I sit here thinking how much courage it takes to live an ordinary life.

—Colum McCann, *Let the Great World Spin*

3
Tornado of Life

Cheryl overdosed on heroin the night before. But that's not the reason she's in the ER late the next day sitting in her gurney, confused.

She woke up this morning so upset to be alive she kicked a wall at the homeless shelter and broke her toe. But that's not why she's in the ER, either.

Something came up a few weeks ago that made her miss her appointment at the methadone clinic. That absence got her kicked out of the clinic for thirty days, or so she said. The withdrawal symptoms made her want to die, and returning to heroin was the easiest solution. But wanting to stop using heroin isn't the reason she's in the ER.

Then her boyfriend died unexpectedly. It wasn't related to their drug use, or so she said. He was in his thirties, an age when hearts don't just give out. He was her love, her reason for getting clean, but he also found her veins. So when she needed heroin after he died, she skin popped.

Angry-looking scars pockmark her arms. She extends them to me and looks away, but neither shame nor infection drove her to the ER late at night.

The police had been called for a disturbance in the shelter that involved Cheryl. She wouldn't shut up, and her mouth earned her a ride to the ER. She didn't want to be here—she made that point loud and painfully clear—yet she complained about the wait to see a doctor. She yelled for attention, and then yelled at the responding nurse that she wanted to be left alone.

When I entered her room and asked what we could do for her, she clammed up.

"Cheryl?"

Her cheeks and jawline were sharp, the sadness in her sea-blue eyes striking. She was thin, too thin, and anxious, practically jumping out of her skin. Symptoms of narcotic withdrawal, or so she said. But these symptoms could also be a separation from, and the need for, a more potent substance: hope.

When I asked Cheryl about what I had read in her medical record—did she want to kill herself—she turned away and didn't answer. I sat there, resisting the urge to fill the silence. Finally, Cheryl took a deep breath and said: "I'm stuck in a tornado of life."

What do you say to someone caught up in the tornado of life, whose problems are so woven into other problems that you're almost afraid to tug at a single thread for fear of everything unraveling?

There was no bottom to her troubles. The plot of Cheryl's story was hard to listen to. I was afraid to ask more questions. Pitted against the "tornado of life," I felt powerless to respond.

Luckily, I recognized that she was telling me a "chaos narrative." The sociologist Arthur Frank frames the pivotal idea of chaos narratives in his book *The Wounded Storyteller: Body, Illness and Ethics*. He suggests that we consider illness experiences and the stories told about them through three different narrative arcs: restitution narratives, quest narratives, and chaos narratives. These terms aren't labels fixed to rigid boxes, but a different set of lenses for examining an experience. Frank claims that the same patient might alternate between these different types of stories during the same illness.

Restitution stories, in broad strokes, are the standard medication commercials on TV. You were living your life in the land of the well when illness suddenly struck. But thanks to the wonders of medical technology, the scientific promise contained in the purple pill, or red or blue, you're cured. Illness becomes a transitory detour from your previous self and your previous life.

Quest stories borrow from the work of Joseph Campbell. It's illness as a journey. You're well, then you depart into the land of the ill. You're initiated into this other place, where you'll face many tests and challenges. The trials you endure—physical, emotional, and social—will transform you. If fortunate to return to the land of the well, you will not be the same person who left. Through illness, you'll discover much about yourself. The experience will inform how you tell the story of your journey. But even those closest to you can't truly fathom the edges of the self you stared into.

Chaos stories are the third of Frank's narratives, and I believe they're the most challenging type of story that patients share in my emergency medicine practice. If a narrative describes a sequence of connected events, then chaos narratives defy such ordering. They signal a complete loss of control. Frank points out that certain troubles run so deep that putting language to these experiences can be difficult, if not impossible. Disorder gives a hurried and harried quality to chaos narratives, as if the person is trying to "catch the suffering in words." It can sound like this: and this happened, and then that happened, and then, and then and then and then.

Was Cheryl's fruitless search for words due to an inability to find the language to express what she was going through? Or, was it that previous experiences with health providers taught her that we couldn't be trusted to hold the messiness of her life in our hands without dropping it, so better say nothing?

Medicine prides itself on restitution narratives and the pretense of control—a romance where problems are managed, cures offered, and suffering remedied. Chaos narratives threaten the safety of this paradigm and cut through clinicians' psychic defenses. They aren't feel-good stories. These unmoored storylines may not only provoke clinicians to interrupt the patient, but also stir their anxieties. Everyone is vulnerable to the tornado of life.

The fundamental challenge when listening to a chaos narrative is sitting with the chaos and not steering the patient away from their feelings. "To deny a chaos story is to deny the person telling the story," wrote Frank, "and people who are being denied cannot be cared for."

Understanding that Cheryl was giving me a chaos narrative clarified my responsibilities. I avoided the reflex to take the wreckage and make a bouquet. I didn't offer balmy optimism, suggest that everything will be okay and you're just going through a tough stretch.

Resisting that impulse was hard, but I took my cue from Frank. "I can't imagine what you're going through," I said, because how could I claim to imagine that which Cheryl can't even put into words. The response to a chaos narrative isn't simplifying what isn't simple or solving the unsolvable, but to sit with the complications and acknowledge that life can be hellish and even hateful. "And I'm not going to pretend that I do."

Cheryl began to cry and tried to laugh the tears away.

"So what's next?" I asked.

A long silence followed.

"Look at me," she said, lifting her arms as if the bruises said everything she couldn't.

"I can see that," I said. "What's next," I asked again. "What happens when you wake up tomorrow? Can you write that line?"

The overwhelming disorder and despair in chaos narratives fix it firmly in the present tense. There's a danger in asking a question that implies that tomorrow can be different from today. But without a sense of empowerment, that change is possible, it's easy to get pulled down by the undertow of troubles that is life for too many people. My persistence walks a tightrope, honoring the severity of her difficulties without giving the impression that I was throwing up my hands in defeat.

Cheryl's hands groped the air, her mouth searching for words. In these situations, it's easy for frustration to creep in. One possible reaction by the listener to this uncomfortable feeling is to feel nothing. There are claims that medical providers suffer from a lack of empathy. But instead of a diminishing or hardening of hearts, I wonder if the problem relates to caring for patients whose needs are overwhelming, ungraspable, and even intimidating, and being at a loss about how to respond.

I understood what was expected of me regarding Cheryl's medical issues. X-ray her toe. Consult psychiatry for her suicide attempt. Take a multidimensional approach to her substance use disorder—aimed toward treatment, overdose prevention, and harm reduction—which would include offering medication-assisted treatment for her withdrawal, counseling with a peer recovery coach, and naloxone training.

Sitting with chaos narratives can be awkward because you must let go and drift with the patient. They're not the stuff of uplifting pharmaceutical ads, which seem to end with smiles, supersaturated sunlight, and the promise of an unpronounceable drug. As the silence grew between us, I fought the pressure to fill it, suggest a remedy of some kind, and move things along. There were other patients to see, other chaos narratives to sit with. But you can't rush chaos narratives regardless of how much you want to. And believe me, I wanted to.

I was surprised by my asking, "Can you write that line?" When Cheryl stopped yelling, I could sense her efforts to disturb the silence. I didn't want to imply that tomorrow would be better, but to acknowledge that tomorrow has weight, that every tomorrow is an achievement.

4
Backstory

Mr. K sits cross-legged on the stretcher, slightly hunched, muscles taut. The cervical collar should be immobilizing his neck, but it lies splayed out in defeat beside him. He's refusing to answer our questions, undress into a gown, or permit us to examine him. "What happened?" I ask, but he's focused on the hospital security officers on either side of his stretcher. His girlfriend called 911 from work after he had called her sounding anxious and panicked and describing a fall. Mr. K served in the military and suffered from post-traumatic stress disorder (PTSD). The EMS (emergency medical services) called to his home met a muscular man who didn't want their help. They found him sitting on the living room floor, breathing fast, trying to calm himself by listening to music. He wouldn't talk to them and refused to be taken to the hospital. There was a disturbing, violent intensity to his resistance. EMS feared for his safety and their own, which is why Mr. K was flanked by police when he arrived in the ER.

The bruise on his forehead is difficult to ignore, a reminder that his behavior might be the result of brain injury, a sign of a concussion or a brain bleed. When there's head trauma, we must also be alert to a possible neck fracture and spinal cord injury. Standard trauma precautions call for neck immobilization in a cervical collar, especially when we can't examine the spine for tenderness or perform a neurological exam. But he won't let us touch his head and neck. He needs a CT (computed tomography) scan of the brain and neck, but that's out of the question.

His voice rises. He demands to be left alone. As more hospital security officers rush into the room, more muscles push through his T-shirt.

If I believe he possesses decision-making capacity, which reflects an understanding of his condition, including the benefits of treatment and the risks of refusal, a respect for patient autonomy means that I permit him to refuse treatment and leave against medical advice. My job involves presenting patients with the best information so they can make well-informed decisions. Ultimately, they're the captains of their bodies. However, when there's a concern for serious, imminent injury, and a patient is either intoxicated, chemically altered, or otherwise thought to lack the capacity to make decisions, clinicians have an obligation to look out for the patient's best interests. A sound idea that isn't much help when figuring out the patient's best interests is part of the problem.

Mr. K still won't permit us near him, and his refusal is growing more adamant. We have a predetermined response to agitated patients. After de-escalation efforts, including non-judgment, respect for their personal space, and clear communication, we move to medications that provide seda-tion for the situational behavior, counter the substances that promote such behavior, or target underlying mental illness if we have that history. Many times, we're address-ing all three possibilities. But if we can't accomplish that, or chemical sedation isn't working, we move to physical restraints.

In a situation such as this, a form of restraint may be the only efficient way to protect patients and staff and to expe-dite any necessary testing, such as a brain CT, to search for a possible brain bleed or other serious medical causes for his behavior. We don't know if his blood sugar is low, if he's under the influence of substances, or whether mental illness is clouding his reasoning. In his present state, he's a possible danger to himself.

But restraint, at its core, leaves a bitter taste. We're infring-ing upon a patient's liberty. And if the patient fights back, the physicality of the methods themselves places patients and staff at risk for harm. You hear yourself using language like "We're doing this for your own good," but the churning in the pit of your stomach is a sign that you need some con-vincing, too.

Mr. K's frustration escalates. The nurse in charge holds the physical restraints in her hand, hinting at what needs to be done. She's waiting for my order and isn't happy with my indecisiveness as tension fills the room. However, Mr. K's agitation seems grounded in a distress that was differ-ent from that of other agitated patients we'd cared for on that shift. In moments such as this one, your moral compass can't always find a true north. You project possibilities based on incomplete information. Only one thing is certain: not making a decision is not an option.

When his girlfriend and his sister arrive, they are understandably upset to see him in this state. I ask if they might talk to him and possibly persuade him to cooperate enough so we can at least examine him. But he won't listen to them, either.

What should I do?

I step into the hallway with Mr. K's girlfriend and sister. I'm aware that leaving the room could be interpreted as an abandonment of my responsibilities and a failure of team leadership, but I feel the need to learn more about him. His girlfriend suspects he might have fallen off a chair while hanging a framed print they recently bought at a local art fair. Mr. K never drinks alcohol or takes drugs, they say. He's a fitness nut. And yes, this behavior is unusual for him, though his sister alludes to previous PTSD episodes that put him in a worried panic, but never this extreme. Never.

I'm lost. I hear him yelling in the room. From their expressions, I sense they're distressed, too.

"Can I ask about his military experience?"

Confusion settles over their faces, as if unclear how it pertains to the problem at hand.

"I'm hoping to learn a little more about his PTSD. How it's impacted his life."

The two women share a look.

"If that's okay? If not, I understand."

There's silence. I strain to read their faces.

Slowly, his girlfriend describes how his PTSD had nothing to do with his military experience. Mr. K had been a victim of rape as a young boy.

My spine turns into cubes of ice.

I look into the room. Muscular men surround his stretcher, threatening to tie him down if he doesn't behave.

What have I done?

I ask everyone to step far away from Mr. K. I'm met with reluctance and shock.

"Please," I say, my tone resolute in defeat. I'm trying to recover my bearings and whatever trust is salvageable with Mr. K.

"Get me out of here," he tells his girlfriend.

I knew certain details about Mr. K's history, but I didn't truly understand his backstory, the desires and fears that animated his behavior. And when I learned about the child-hood trauma that led to his PTSD, and recognized my role in his terror, I became ashamed of myself.

After I ask the security officers to leave, a quiet sits over the room. Mr. K meets my eyes. I can barely look at him. He allows me to explain my concern for a neck fracture, a brain bleed, or some other injury. But I don't believe he's listening. Besides, how should he judge the possible risks of leaving after enduring the real risks of our concern? He agrees to let me examine his head and neck, but he pulls away as soon as I touch his skin. He's done. Let me go, he says, his voice assertively apologetic.

There were no CT scans of the brain and neck. No physical exam. And no real clarity on what had happened at home. I'd shattered his trust. Once that happens, it might be patched together, but never fully repaired. I've learned this weaker version might be functional, but rarely can it support the full weight of clinician and patient moving forward side by side.

I apologize one last time. I run through a list of concerning symptoms that might prompt a return visit and reiterate that we want him back should he change his mind. After this experience, I wonder if he'll ever set foot in another ER. His girlfriend and sister nod appreciatively. They'll keep a close eye on him. But we all know the real suffering has already happened. Mr. K pulls himself off the stretcher. I'm startled, embarrassed even, when he lifts his head halfway while tucking in his shirt and says, "Thank you."

Coda

Mr. K's emotional state was treated as pathology that demanded a response, rather than evidence in a narrative that needed further investigation. Despite all the harms that take place in hospitals, ones less frequently addressed are narrative errors. I've noticed this tendency in our monthly morbidity and mortality (M&M) conferences, where we review cases to improve system processes or medical knowledge. I consider myself very fortunate to work in an academic department with brilliant colleagues who not only know the latest medical literature but do groundbreaking research. Not infrequently, the root of the problem in these cases isn't a lack of knowledge, but smart physicians who just got the story wrong.

The narrative scholar Kathryn Montgomery said it beautifully: "Clinicians . . . work to perfect the maps of illness, but each patient, each instance of illness, is unchartered territory."

A physician faced with an agitated patient with signs of head trauma won't be faulted for using some form of judicious restraint to accomplish the necessary testing to rule out a potential life-threatening head injury or medical catastrophe as an explanation for such behavior. However, a justified action doesn't necessarily mean it's the right or the best option.

Rigorous research studies lead to clinical guidelines and protocols to ensure that we meet standards of quality. We find great comfort in such recommendations—who doesn't welcome a well-paved road with clearly marked signs? But that comfort is fraught with risk if we steer patients onto these roads even if their story is ill fit for it.

I can't break down the shift in perspective, identify specific clues that alerted me that something was amiss. I recognized a feeling, a pressure that arises when I'm writing and a story is disorganized, not going anywhere. This clinical situation felt like this impasse, as was the temptation to push forward and do something. I've since learned the question, "What's next?" begins with taking a step back and asking, "How did I get here, and why?" What's the central conflict? Can I identify the forces motivating Mr. K and myself? Sometimes, the urge to act in the patient's best interests begins by trying to understand the inner experience of another.

5
Why Medicine Needs More Not-Knowing

Let's consider Jill L, a well-dressed woman who comes to a busy, inner-city ER late one Saturday night with vague symptoms that include chest pain and shortness of breath. She's easily the best-dressed and best-smelling person in the entire ER, and that includes the staff. The young ER doc isn't that concerned about anything serious at first, but something doesn't sit right, and he returns several times to clarify her symptoms. He's left with little to latch onto except chest pain and shortness of breath, so that's where he goes.

Could this be a possible heart attack? It's unlikely. She's in her mid-thirties with no cardiac risk factors. Maybe a blood clot shot to her lung? The workup stretches through the night, and yet she sleeps undeterred by the tumult around her. When daylight comes, and he apologizes for being unable to find an explanation for her symptoms, she knuckles sleep from her eyes, offers a smile, and says how much she appreciates his efforts.

The young ER doc is diligent, courteous, and devoid of any imagination. He never thinks to ask why? Why did this impeccably dressed woman change obvious evening plans to come to this ER at this time of night for what sounds like vague concerns, when there is nothing vague about her? Her eye-catching diamond ring and wedding band didn't spark questions. Sleeping alongside these grumpy, snoring strangers on an uncomfortable stretcher seemed preferable to curling up at home in her comfortable bed with her spouse or partner, who isn't here.

If he'd asked, she might have told him the real reason for her visit—hours earlier, before all the testing. For years, she'd endured physical and emotional abuse from her husband, and she'd finally, finally had enough.

The doctor who rushed to find the answer rather than acknowledge the nagging uncertainty, who chased her symptoms but failed to engage with the landscape of her story, was a young me at the start of my medical career.

In his book *A Fortunate Man*, a portrait of a country doctor in rural England, John Berger writes: "Landscapes can be deceptive. Sometimes a landscape seems to be less a setting for the life of its inhabitants than a curtain behind which their struggles, achievements, and accidents take place."

Berger challenges our common understanding of landscapes. He provokes the reader to consider how we navigate these physical and emotional spaces, this magnificent, mysterious, and sometimes treacherous terrain hidden from others or unrecognizable as a space that requires attention. I believe these challenges aren't commonly addressed in medical training, because they require a critical concept that one might consider antithetical to medical practice—"not-knowing."

I borrowed this notion of "not-knowing" from the writer Donald Barthelme's essay of the same name. In this essay, Barthelme describes the act of writing, and the creative arts in general, as a process of dealing with not-knowing. The writer is someone who, when embarking upon a messy task, doesn't know what to do. Problems are crucial to not-knowing, and not-knowing is crucial to art. Embracing problems is not only critical to the creative process, Barthelme states, but the seriousness of the artist is defined by the seriousness of the problems they take on.

Working with patient stories is a creative investigation. It requires a sensitivity to what's missing in the landscape or what's hidden. From the position of "not-knowing" we remain open when symptoms don't make sense and find comfort in that openness. It sounds counterintuitive, but we need more not-knowing because medicine has an uncertainty problem. In 1989, Dr. Jerome Kassirer, former editor of the *New England Journal of Medicine*, wrote, "Absolute certainty in diagnosis is unattainable, no matter how much information we gather, how many observations we make and how many tests we perform."

Uncertainty is a cognitive challenge that's felt in the body, and it doesn't feel good. Personally, uncertainty can feel like anything from a mild allergic reaction to a panic attack. A quick fix for the discomfort that comes with uncertainty is certainty—or at least its pretense. Under the pressures of clinical practice, our instinct is to reach for more data, which usually means more diagnostic testing. Today, medicine doesn't suffer for a lack of knowledge. Researchers do an impressive job of generating data. One study reported that seventy-five clinical trials and eleven systematic reviews are published every day. But such abundance poses challenges, including keeping up, making sense of it all, and separating the signal from the noise.

So majestic are these mountains of information, the limitations are not immediately apparent. The problem isn't uncertainty, per se, but the clinician's relationship to it. As we saw with Jill L, more data doesn't promise more certainty if it's in the service of the wrong questions. Even the best data gleaned from studying populations of patients is helpful only once I've defined the problem for which this data applies. It can be the wrong tool for providers unprepared for the complexity, ambiguity, instability, and value conflicts that are often the source of real anxieties in medical practice. A strict focus on data can even be dangerous if it blinds us to other lines of inquiry, and distracts us from wading into other forms of data buried in stories. Taking this path into stories never encountered before can be a source of discomfort, too. It doesn't promise answers, but it's often the only chance for us to discover the very thing we didn't know we were looking for.

Barthelme writes about how problems present opportunities to push our thinking into unanticipated directions; without problems, there would be no invention. With Jill L, I felt stuck, which produced a boxed-in panic because being stuck in medicine can imply failure. This message was drilled into me early in my medical training. A fourth-year medical student shared this bit of wisdom at the beginning of my third-year clerkships that he learned from his previous year on the wards: "You can be wrong, but never in doubt."

Through the lens of not-knowing, we have permission to be stuck. We welcome being stuck. It might be the only clue that we're onto something, our inner alarm system quietly screaming for us to pay attention.

Developing comfort with uncertainty is hard when physicians are incentivized for having the answers, not for owning up to what they don't know. Outcome metrics don't reward physicians for not-knowing. However, when there's a disconnect between the stories we tell and stories people experience, and a patient's deepest troubles are often found between the lines, in the silences and oblique language that signals evasion, fear, or mistrust, the ability to sit with uncertainty must be encouraged and valued.

I wasn't comfortable admitting my confusion to Jill L, to confess all that I didn't know. How did I change my focus and learn about the real reason for Jill L's visit? I didn't. She took pity on me, or so I believe. In the morning, before discharging her home, I asked whether there was anyone we might call to come to get her. She made a passing comment about not wanting to contact her husband. Even I picked up on that elliptical phrasing—what she wasn't saying but wanted me to hear. She swung the door wide open as far as it could go, and all I had to do was curl into a ball of shame and roll inside.

Not-knowing should not be confused with ignorance. It's not lack of knowledge or poor application of knowledge. I should know the correct antibiotics for treating hospital-acquired pneumonia. I better have a ruptured aortic aneurysm in the forefront of my mind when considering an older patient with the sudden onset of abdominal pain. Not-knowing begins with a solid foundation of medical knowledge. Without that, it's hard to know what you don't know.

Not knowing is a muscle that can become stronger and stabilized only through training and interrogation of our thinking process, starting with the decisions we make even before we think we're making decisions. For example, why do we choose specific details in a patient's story to focus on—like chest pain and difficulty breathing in Jill L's case—and not others? The story I created about Jill L was very different from the one she was telling.

A richly documented history of symptoms and past medical problems can still miss the troubles and needs plaguing a particular person at a moment in their lives. Listening to a story is a different exercise than listening to a patient's symptoms. It requires many of the same muscles as creative writing. When writing stories, you move into what Eudora Welty calls "open spaces." You're aware of characters, the choices they have to make, and how the stakes can amplify very quickly. You're also sensitive to the narrative directions not taken. The elements that don't belong or make sense. The dialogue that takes you by surprise. By thinking this way with Welty's open spaces, the physician can resist the urge to impose the wrong structure, a false ending, or yield a quick judgment.

Looking back, I recognize how much of my conversation with Jill L was subtext, and I hadn't paid attention to what was between the lines, the gaps in her story. Not only didn't I know where to look, I wasn't savvy enough to realize there was a curtain behind which I had to look. Patients don't always share their grave concerns directly. They'll tell stories and expect physicians to probe and pick up on their feelings of fear, anger, or anxiety and ask them questions.

Story isn't the vehicle toward a diagnosis, it's the destination. And when a patient's story becomes unwieldy or doesn't point to an obvious solution, it's easy enough to engage with patients at the level of story. "I understand, you have chest pain, your stomach hurts, your feet tingle, you're weak and tired, you have headaches and body aches, you have a rash that went away, your stomach is bloated, and your urine smells strange. Take me through your day today, and what you were doing and what exactly was bothering you that made you say enough, I have to go to the ER."

Narrative is an "invitation to problem finding, not a lesson in problem solving," says the narrative scholar Jerome Bruner. "It is deeply about plight, about the road rather than about the inn to which it leads."

Story is about trouble. Something has gone awry. And isn't that why people are so interested in stories about illness? What's gone awry isn't only our bodies. There are other threats in play: our identity, our relationship with our bodies, our conception of ourselves, and our relationships with others. A common thread that runs through various unrelated complaints is a patient's fear of losing control. Story provides a landscape where they can express and validate their experiences.

For all the pronouncements about technological inno-
vation disrupting and transforming medicine, I believe the
platform of story—patients telling stories to physicians and
physicians telling stories back to patients—is a powerful tool
for dealing with a critical challenge in medicine—working
through uncertainty. Without story at its core, medicine
can't practice responsible, evidence-based care.

So how do we cultivate a physician's comfort with uncertainty? In practical terms, not-knowing asks that physicians
think more like artists, those who are experts in the practice of uncertainty, and focus more on process. Making art
reflects our beliefs and how we think about the world. Whatever is produced represents an accounting of our mind at
work. Process receives less attention in medicine than outcomes. Outcome measurements are important, but I fear that
the emphasis on results has diminished the value of other
practices foundational to medicine but harder to quantify.

We'd like believe we're savvy to what's going on in our
minds, that our decisions are a linear string of conscious
thoughts. However, my impressions and beliefs often appear
out of the dark quiet, a product of insecurities as much as
reason. I must recognize when there are curtains and find
methods for throwing them back.

Barthelme writes about the purposes of art, but he speaks
to our work in medicine, too: that art is a true account of the
activity of the mind; art thinks ever of the world; and art's
project, ultimately, is to better the world. This is a difficult
task, but taking on this challenge appeals to the seriousness

of the artist in all of us, especially when we're wearing a white coat.

When I was caring for Jill L, I was aware of the prevalence of interpersonal violence (IPV), how it permeates all socioeconomic classes. Screening for IPV wasn't standard back then, but I knew many victims present with vague complaints, that they often visit a healthcare setting multiple times before their troubles come to light. I was well aware that a significant percentage of victims won't come forward on their own, but will open up when asked directly by clinicians. My problem wasn't "knowing" but "not-knowing": failing to recognize the landscape and the importance of traveling it.

Imagination is necessary to understand another human, not only what's going on in their story but also what could or should be. My growth as a physician has been, and continues to be, interwoven with my growth as a writer. Writing isn't a linear process. It often requires detours and tangents to discover what you're writing about. I'm inspired by creative artists like the poet Mark Doty, who describes uncertainty as a good thing, how in "in any process of inquiry, our uncertainty is our ally." The ability to welcome uncertainty as a place of unfolding possibility is a critical part of doctoring, too. Sometimes, the questions we ask attest to our clinical acumen as much as if not more than the answers we offer.

6
Ambassador to Nightmares

I'm a physician, a husband and dad, a guy who tries to live by the golden rule. But sometimes what I do unto others is escort them into a nightmare, plunging families into the darkest depths with the news I must give them.

A case from earlier years stands out. Mary would have been starting college in a few weeks. Instead, the car in which she was a passenger collided with a truck. My emergency department team couldn't resuscitate her. Right after we called the time of death, a nurse gasped. With a shaking hand, she pointed to Mary's cell, which we had removed from her jeans when we cut off her clothes. "Where are you!!" the text message said. It was from Dad.

The nurse, also a mother and a wife, excused herself.

Later, I'm sitting in the windowless family room packed with a chair, two small couches, and space enough for knees, telling Mary's parents that their daughter is dead, acutely aware of my role in their nightmare.

Nightmares are vivid, disturbing dreams that elicit fear, anxiety, and sadness. They can jerk us out of sleep to escape the perceived danger or unpleasantness. I traffic in nightmares made real, sit with families as they shake themselves in a desperate attempt to prove they're not awake. The emotional burden of talking with them is compounded by the fact that my son will be driving in a few short years. When my grief touches theirs, it's as a physician and as a parent. However, it's a vicarious version of grief; a sudden peek behind the lines of psychic defenses that usually protect me from the darkest corners of my imagination.

I strive to balance sympathy against the hardness of clarity, sensitive to the absolute weight of my words and how they will land on those who receive them. I'm supposed to prepare them for the news to come, but it's all horrific. Crushed car. No seat belt. No airbags to soften the impact of this story. The moment of first hearing the news becomes its own collision. For a split-second time stops and the oxygen is sucked from the room.

I use the word "died," not "passed" or "couldn't bring her back" or some other euphemism ripe for misinterpretation. I'm sorry. My chest aches as I watch their eyes glaze over and their faces crinkle with disbelief. I'm so, so sorry for your loss. Vacant stares, then tears. But it hasn't fully hit them yet. I wait. The questions will come when they're ready. What happened? Why? How could she die? How? The family shakes off everything I say as if begging me to change my answers. Any answer will do as long as their daughter is alive.

In this highly concentrated moment, I may catch most of Elisabeth Kübler-Ross's stages of grief—denial, anger, bargaining, and depression—flashing like a disco ball spinning off its axis.

If I could possess magical powers, I'd use it to write a different story about their daughter. But such speculation, I realize, is a selfish exercise, a weak balm for my discomfort. Their nightmare is a solid piece. I can't find a single seam or joint in this narrative where I can insert hope. It's hard to meet their eyes. Especially now, as they size me up suspiciously, from my button-down shirt down to my shoes. "Could a better doctor have saved our daughter?"

We're strangers thrust together by cruel circumstance. Without a shared history, there's no bank of trust to draw on. The outcome was sealed before Mary arrived in the emergency department. But when your job requires making quick, life-and-death decisions based on limited and often imperfect information, it's impossible not to question yourself if you care enough.

"Why couldn't you save her?" says Mary's sister, tossing in a few insults under her breath. "Isn't this a hospital?"

I can't argue. Though Mary suffered severe multisystem trauma with no signs of life at the scene of the collision, that doesn't necessarily dampen the appetite for miracles. Studies show the public is overly optimistic when it comes to predicting recovery after cardiopulmonary resuscitation. The media contributes to the misinformation. People on television shows whose hearts stop recover more often than in real life. Often they wake up, without neurological damage, as if there's little difference between a brief excursion with death and a deep sleep.

I give Mary's sister room for her torment. I recognize her pain, though I could never imagine it.

That's why I never use scripted language like "I know what you're going through," because nothing could be further from the truth. All grief is specific and private and tangled up in relationships. Mary had been trying to get her life together, her father says. No, she was getting her life together, her mother insists.

The mood shifts in the room. I no longer see judgment signaled in the family's lost, faraway looks; what is silently communicated is an altogether different wish. Please, please leave us alone. I've done everything in my power, and it wasn't nearly enough. The small couch they're scrunched into has become an island and I'm no longer useful to the family. Death from trauma such as car crashes—events that are sudden, unexpected, premature, violent, and potentially avoidable—is particularly jarring for those left behind. I'm grateful for the social worker squeezed into the room with us. What comfort can I offer when a hybrid poet, psychologist, and high priest of grief wouldn't reach the depths of what they're feeling?

I've witnessed grief so aggressive that I feared for my safety. The adult daughter of a patient once charged at me, ready to hit me, only to collapse at my feet. Another time an adult son grabbed my white coat, pulled me out of my chair and, refusing to accept what I was saying, demanded that I leave the family room and do more for his now dead parent. I've also sat before dull nods, as if the family had been awaiting this heartbreak but didn't know when it would appear. And there was a family relieved to be free of their estranged father, but upset because this swindler had had the last laugh, sticking them with a hospital bill and the cost of a funeral they could never afford.

There isn't a "right" or "expected" response at moments like these. The families are the settlers in this unbearable nightmare. Who am I to judge whether their emotions and experiences animating those feelings are appropriate?

The medical literature is rich with conceptual thinking on breaking bad news, along with protocols and communication interventions that give guidance for doctors in training as well as physicians in clinical practice. As a medical student many years ago, I didn't receive any formal education. That wasn't uncommon at the time. These days, it's often delivered through teaching modules bearing the name "breaking bad news" or "difficult conversations."

Despite the best efforts to study, understand, and train for these encounters in emergency medicine, plus excellent analyses and studies dating back many decades, actually doing them never feels right. Telling a family about the death of a loved one who had endured chronic problems and had been in and out of the hospital is hard enough. But Mary's day began as any other. Her parents expected her home in the evening. Until they received the call, they had enjoyed the luxury of being upset at her for staying out so late.

Families remember these moments. The impact of a physician's words can last a lifetime. Since I'm meeting families like Mary's for the first time, my communication skills ride a tightrope over a perilous abyss. What I say shapes their impression of this moment. If I give them this news with diligence and attentiveness, perhaps they'll understand that our efforts to resuscitate Mary, despite the tragic ending, were carried out the same way.

In situations like these, the family members become victims themselves, and researchers have recommended they be considered patients for the immediate time, suggesting that skilled interventions may help reduce what are called "pathologic" grief responses. For example, complicated bereavement and post-traumatic stress disorder are particular risks for the loved ones of people who die in car crashes. However, I presume other scenarios where death is sudden and unexpected must be equally destabilizing. The hardest part of being an ambassador to nightmares isn't leading people to this lost place, but leaving them there.

Thinking of family and loved ones as patients fortifies my commitment to this process and highlight the limits of what's under my control. But new challenges emerged during the COVID-19 pandemic. It didn't matter whether the death was directly related to SARS-CoV-2 or some other cause. Families weren't allowed into hospitals during the pandemic, which raised the degree of difficulty of these already difficult discussions.

Before COVID-19, experts in breaking bad news emphasized the importance of having these nuanced and often complicated conversations face-to-face. Using the phone or other forms of technology was discouraged, and considered only as a method of last resort. A 2019 pre-COVID incident caused a media stir and highlighted the challenges of communication mediated through technology.

A seventy-eight-year-old patient with chronic lung disease and difficulty breathing received his poor prognosis from a robot—a physician who appeared on a screen that rolled up to his hospital bed. This event sparked conversations that ranged from the importance and shortfalls of telemedicine, how we square technology with intimacy and the human touch, the generational differences in our relationships and comfort with technology, and whether we're blaming the screen for the physician's screen-side manner. COVID-19 raised the anxiety ante for those of us serving as ambassadors to nightmares, expected to deliver news into a space without walls.

During the pandemic, I came to miss that small family room. Tighter than most walk-in closets, the space may feel like a cocoon from which you never want to leave or an oven that you can't escape quickly enough. But this family room provides structure and a semblance of control. I can measure a family's facial expressions, how they look to each other, or hang their heads; whether they're ready for more information or need time to absorb the news and reclaim their bearings. I can read whether a light touch of their hand is needed or appropriate. Even if I can't rescue families from their island of grief, the undeniable connection between humans is most evident during shared sorrow, and their proximity allowed me to be a more responsible and compassionate steward.

I felt unmoored as an ambassador to nightmares early in the new COVID-19 world. Alma, a nursing home resident with COVID, came to the ER in respiratory distress and quickly fell into cardiac arrest. There was a confusing advance directive. Resuscitative measures failed, and she died. When I spoke to the daughter over the phone, I learned her mother had been frail with many medical problems, but from the chatter in the background over speakerphone, I could tell they never expected she would die now. I strained to make out their concerns. I couldn't tell who was crying and who was talking to whom. The daughter was speaking for the family, but her husband was now shepherding questions. He said she was understandably quite upset and it was better that I talk with him. Was I still on speaker phone? He was whispering now. I expressed sympathy—for his mother-in-law's death, and the distant, awkward manner in which I had to break the news.

If I served as a personal escort into grief for Mary's family, with Alma's it felt like I was operating a drone from miles away.

Months later, when restrictions on family members eased and they were allowed into the ER for end-of-life situations, I became reacquainted with this space and discovered there were corners I could no longer reach. A woman in her fifties died unexpectedly and her daughter rushed to the hospital wearing the uniform from her job at a local fast food restaurant. She's college-aged, only she's caring for her young siblings and a father who can't work owing to traumatic brain injury. I strained to read and respond to her face hidden behind a mask. I didn't know whether my sympathy would reach her from behind my mask and goggles. She cried silently. I was grateful to be in a position to give her a box of tissues, to sit with her. Her hard life had suddenly become a nightmare. Before, when she didn't know what to do, she always asked her mother. Tough beyond her years, she tried to smile away the tears.

Inside this room, the nightmare was real, but she didn't have to take it into the world, not yet anyway. For a final minute or two, she could let the mask dangle from an ear and breathe. The social worker would help her as much as he could, calling her aunts, telling her family, making funeral arrangements. Eventually, she'd need to step into the hallway.

I've noticed how people often blink a few times when they emerge from the family room and brush shoulders with others going about their day. The sounds of normalcy must feel loud and unbearable. When I finish with Mary's family, the light in the hospital hallway feels too bright. I want to yell at two nurses innocently laughing as they return from break. I can't imagine what laughter sounds like to Mary's family or any family told that their loved one is unexpectedly dead.

Mary's father calls after me. He looks me up and down, runs his fingers through his hair. Then he shakes my hand, his grip firm, as if to brace from collapsing. Words feel like the husks of empty seeds in my mouth. I match his grip—as a physician, as a father, as a man struggling with his own emotions.

I treasure that handshake with Mary's father. So much is communicated in that simple gesture—shared sorrow, suffering, empathy, and an understanding that this moment is over and it's time to depart. Ending a phone call, meanwhile, is abrupt and absolute. To date, technology presents no closure surrogate that could replace a handshake or that slight, comforting tap on the shoulder.

Escorting those left behind, parent or spouse or sibling or friend, into a world that most of us can't even imagine might be the toughest task in emergency medicine. Sometimes I worry that a death in the family might signify a death of the family. I think every emergency physician dreams of an idealized future where scientific and social advances render the position "ambassador to nightmares" obsolete. Until that time, I will continue to learn how to deliver bombshell news with compassion and care. That process requires a degree of openness and a willingness to be vulnerable. There's no hiding behind a white coat. Through the years it hasn't become easier. And I hope it never does.

7
Catheters

I ask the nursing home resident to explain the indwelling catheter in her bladder placed during her last hospital admission weeks earlier.

"How should I know? You go into the hospital and come out with these things."

8

When Loneliness Is an Emergency

Iona Potatov is a broken and lonely cab driver reeling from sorrow. Earlier in the week, his son fell suddenly ill and died. If Iona came to the hospital, his chief complaint on his ER chart might read: "To whom shall I tell my grief?"

Iona is the protagonist in Anton Chekhov's 1886 short story "Misery," but his experience of anguish, his private and overwhelming despair, is often at the heart of what ails many of my ER patients. Chekhov takes the reader on an interior journey into one man's distress, makes the pressure of Iona's loneliness palpable and his hunger for connection raw. I reread "Misery" often—shorter than most articles in medical journals, it's arguably more clinically significant.

"To whom shall I tell my grief?" may sound strange to our ears. But when the answer is "No one," it cuts across time and place and feels achingly current.

Like Iona, many of my patients suffer for want of what Abraham Maslow considers the most basic of needs—warmth, food, shelter, security, and a sense of connection.

We find Iona at twilight, grief ridden and trying to work. Business is slow. Snowflakes swirl about the streetlamps and cover his body as he sits in a horse-drawn carriage. When he finds passengers, he strains to talk about his dead son. Only, he doesn't find a sympathetic ear. He endures indifference, insults, and even a cruel whack on the back of his neck. The streets are crowded, and yet not a single person can be bothered to hear about his misery that's "immense, beyond all bounds."

Approximately one in three older Americans report feeling lonely—and isolation is associated with a range of long-term health consequences, including functional decline and an increased risk for heart disease and stroke. A review found that individuals without meaningful social relationships are twice as likely to die. The mortality risk for people lacking social connection compares with cigarette smoking and is twice as dangerous as obesity. Loneliness is a significant and growing public health problem in other countries as well. In the UK, the government went so far as to appoint a Minister of Loneliness.

It's hard to admit to loneliness. In his book, *Together: The Healing Power of Human Connection in a Sometimes Lonely World*, Dr. Vivek Murthy, the nineteenth and twenty-first surgeon general of the United States, wrote how when people feel lonely, there is a paradoxical inclination to withdraw from groups instead of approaching them. Our shame and fear trigger self-doubt, which further lowers our self-esteem and discourages us from reaching out. This vicious loop, says Dr. Murthy so astutely, can "drive us further inward and away from the relationships we need most."

If there's a modern telling of "Misery," and Iona Potatov presents to the emergency department because he has nowhere else to turn, would pride force him to seek refuge behind physical complaints like chest pain, weakness, dizziness, or not eating? Would I pick up on any shame and embarrassment, hints that I need to look beneath the facade of these more acceptable medical conditions for the truly worrisome social and health problem—loneliness? If not, and I recruit blood work, EKGs, even imaging to this investigation of his chief complaints, his workup would seem appropriate at a surface level, even though I failed to provide what he most desperately needed. Missing his cry for connection could leave him feeling more alone. Iona Potatov may think twice the next time he aches to reach out.

There are times, especially when I'm working overnight, when decision-making requires more than an interpretation of what symptoms mean to include what they're hiding. Does chest pain imply pain in the chest, raising concerns for a heart attack, for example? Or does it veil other needs, such as a warm bed, relief from the streets, a reprieve from stressful living situations, unbearable anxiety, or a yearning to speak about the death of a son? I see Iona Potatov in the mother complaining of abdominal pain who just buried her second son from an accidental overdose; this time, it was fentanyl. Before her, there was a young woman with a terrible headache whose son recently died of cancer. There's a man in his thirties who lost both parents to COVID-19, worried that he might be infected, too. But he doesn't describe a cough, fever, abdominal pain, diarrhea, or a change in smell. Instead, he spends most of the time grieving, lamenting how he couldn't see them in the hospital, how they died days apart and alone.

"To whom shall I tell my grief?"

I'd like to believe that whenever Iona, or someone like him, comes to the ER, he'll find providers to talk with him "properly, with deliberation." But there's a chance he might leave as profoundly disappointed in my response as he was in the others.

Emergency departments shoulder the acute burden of care for insured and uninsured populations. At these hubs for complex diagnostic workups for patients with multiple complicated medical problems, patients with less acute-sounding issues may receive less of our time and deliberation. Juggling many sick and injured patients simultaneously requires allocating attention, but concluding that I need to direct my attention with more sensitivity is to miss the point.

Sure, time is scarce; electronic medical records are cumbersome; health systems are in chaos. I believe another culprit is responsible for our misdirected attention, and we own it. In his book *Ways of Seeing*, John Berger said, "We only see what we look at. To look is an act of choice." Framed in this manner, what I value as important is on trial. My attention becomes subject to judgment.

If Iona sat before me in a hospital gown and his story unfolded slowly or took detours, would I direct my attention appropriately? Would I wait to learn that if his "heart were to burst and his misery to flow out, it would flood the whole world"? Or, would I interrupt him, as studies found, at around twenty-three seconds? This isn't a theoretical question. Stories are at the heart of emergency care, caring for lives troubled by various scales of misfortune that have little to do with disease or injury. When a patient's suffering far exceeds my capacity to help, it produces a despair in me that, in a subconscious move of self-protection, might put at a distance the very patients I need to draw closer to.

When Iona returns with his little mare to his lodging, a flophouse, he finds snoring men strewn about the floors and benches, but not a single person willing to listen to him. He wants—he needs—to talk about how his son fell ill, how he suffered, his last words, Iona's trip to the hospital to collect his son's clothes.

At the story's end, Iona puts on his coat and visits his mare in the stables. Watching her munch on hay—he hadn't earned enough that evening to buy her oats—Iona opens his heart.

"Now, suppose you had a little colt, and you were own mother to that little colt . . . And all at once that same little colt went and died . . . You'd be sorry, wouldn't you . . . ?"

Chekhov ends the story with the mare munching, listening and breathing on her master's hand.

The mare knows to breathe on Iona's hands.

Dr. John Lantos has written about how we see ourselves more easily in stories, learning "not just what we ought to aspire to, but how easy it is to fail to reach those aspirations." Iona deserves what many patients crave as well: not only medical expertise and technology, but recognition, dignity, and the warmth of a fellow human. If Iona should come to the ER one night and ask, "To whom shall I tell my grief?" I must close the curtain, pull up a chair, and say, "Me. I'm here. I'm all yours."

9
Trust as Protection

I stepped through the sliding glass doors of my hospital's emergency department and found my previously used surgical mask in a paper bag with my name scribbled on the outside. I breathed deeply and wrinkled my nose at the smell. It's a stale, tired scent, unrecognizable and unpleasant.

Hellos from the nurses behind the newly erected makeshift Plexiglas distracted me from the smell, as did the friendly greetings exchanged with docs, physician assistants, techs, unit secretaries, social workers, interpreters, housekeepers, and the others I've worked alongside for years. But there were gasps of astonishment, too. I smiled bashfully at their shock. The night before, I'd shaved my beard to ensure a tight seal between my skin with the N95 mask. My face burned from a clean shave for the first time in thirty years. The cloth covering my bare cheeks couldn't hide how exposed I felt, like a turtle without its shell.

Sure, I was apprehensive and stressed. By stepping into the ER, I was at considerable risk for being exposed to and infected by the COVID-19 virus, at the time a new, relatively unknown infection wreaking havoc around the globe and now knocking on our door. The dubious state of personal protection stoked my anxiety further. Imagine my surprise to discover the mask-smell, high in my nostrils, was washed away by this banter with my coworkers, that I felt safest at work.

I couldn't make sense of the response from leaders who should have been bastions of guidance and support. One day we were told that providers must scrupulously don an N95 mask, face shield, portable gown, and gloves. Then the shortage of personal protective equipment somehow altered scientific evidence, and the CDC believed that surgical masks, which fit like a pair of old khakis, should be more than adequate. When stockpiles of personal protection equipment resembled the empty toilet paper aisle in grocery stores, I anticipated an announcement that they had good evidence, excellent evidence, the best evidence ever, that taking a marker and drawing an N95 mask on your face is just as effective as wearing an actual surgical mask. But it would be best if you used a permanent marker.

We were instructed to reuse the N95 and surgical masks, which took on a mysterious odor after a day or two. I soon identified that smell. It was mistrust.

In times of crisis, transparency and trust are essential. But when trust becomes a resource as scarce as personal protective equipment, it can't be manufactured or extended beyond its intended terms of use. Trust is difficult to describe and put into words, but you know when it's missing. You feel abandoned, disappointed, and pissed off. I also became grateful for the trust I hadn't recognized before, which explains my comfort working in the ER at the start of the pandemic. It meant being surrounded by people I trust inherently.

If there's a group of people prepared for the uncertainty that surrounded this coronavirus, it was the emergency staff I worked hand-and-glove with, people with big personalities, bigger hearts, and the resilience of Gumby. Facing bodies and lives in crisis is part of our regular day. So is responding quickly with limited and conflicting information at our fingertips. Since testing for COVID-19 was as scarce as personal protective equipment, we couldn't always see our foe. We had no choice but to assume every patient harbored the virus. Caring for our patients while ensuring that we stay safe and healthy demanded that we care for each other.

ER staff are practiced in doing more with less. Even before COVID-19, this space buckled from the strain of serving two masters: meeting the growing needs of communities while working as part of a stressed hospital. In the beginning, I wondered about preparedness, especially when the physical space felt like a confusion of design and purpose, a blend of high technology and elementary school lunchroom. It boasted monitors, CT scanners, MRI suites, and a cardiac catheterization lab, while strewn along shelves and countertops sat rows of brown paper bags in which we stored our multiuse masks and face shields.

It might sound counterintuitive to confess that I felt safest and most protected in the ER. Protection came in the form of the talented, tenacious, and compassionate people who make the ER hum. We'd been through so much together, albeit on a much smaller scale. We were well practiced in personal risk and having each other's back, frequently on the receiving end of violence, verbal abuse, and infections.

The trust that sustained me was forged from years of working together. We shared triumphs, endured troubles, and exposed our vulnerabilities. I've been at my best with my colleagues and at my worst. As the second surge mounted in November 2020, I was at my worst. Many of us were still feeling the strain of the first wave when this surge brought suffering and dying COVID-19 patients and all the other people who stayed away from seeing their doctors, or vice versa. Patients with ignored strokes, heart attacks, poorly controlled diabetes, infections, and mental health disorders. And there was the trauma, the substance use, the diseases of despair. The lack of inpatient beds due to prolonged hospitalizations from COVID-19 meant more inpatients boarded in the ER. Homeless patients with mild or asymptomatic COVID-19 also remained in the ER until we could find them appropriate housing.

Once, when finishing up after a frustrating overnight shift, an ER tech confronted me. They had been talking, she said. They'd noticed a change in me and they didn't like it. Her message was clear: Knock it off. I began explaining my personal troubles, but quickly stopped. We were all going through difficult times. They needed me to be less serious and short-tempered, and would it kill me to show a hint of my old sense of humor?

We rib each other incessantly, teasing built out of affection and respect. When you bust on the unit secretary about her overhead call for the owner of the red Toyota to please move their "cah," you're really saying I'm glad we're working together this shift. That moment of tough love from this crackerjack tech shook me to the core, and explains why I trust these people in a crisis. Such brutally honest feedback has made me a better doctor and hopefully a better person.

When you joke together and hold each other accountable, it's easier to deal with the absurdity of guidelines that possessed a whiff of fiction to them. For example, early criteria for deciding whether a patient should be suspected of having SARS-CoV-2 included "prolonged, unprotected close contact with a patient with symptomatic, confirmed COVID-19." But the lack of testing was a huge problem at the time.

When the masks I was expected to wear and wear out took on a gamey odor from so much use, I was vitalized by working alongside such smart, strong, and funny colleagues. Sure, we knocked heads. We also tied and secured the backs of each other's gowns and diligently checked for gaps in protection that we all knew was more porous than we'd like. We reminded each other to drink enough fluids. And don't forget to eat, too. We checked in and asked how we were doing. We made it through that difficult time through trust and coming together. Fortunately, that's something we've been working on for years.

10
Upside Down

Pushed through the ER entrance on a gurney. A voice directed the medics to a treatment bay. Hands removed my shirt and attached wires to my chest and finger. Monitors stood at my head, passing judgments. I eyed the fast heart rate and low oxygen level in my blood as if the numbers belonged to someone else. In Providence, Rhode Island, where I'm an ER doc, these monitors are my allies. Now, I was in a North Carolina ER, sweat-soaked, breathing hard, caked in vomit, and my scalp a bloody mess.

Doctors and nurses spoke to me and across me. Visual noise competed for my attention: scrubs, white coats, medic uniforms, and in the distance, police and patients on gurneys. My throbbing head was alert to strange background chatter—alarms and urgent hospital-wide announcements, including code words for a life that needs saving and a Jell-O spill that requires mopping.

My EKG showed an injury pattern seen with people having an acute heart attack. I tried to inform my fretting doctors the ugly-looking EKG was better than it once was. It's hard to reconcile the past when the disorienting present feels like a carnival.

That evening, I had torpedoed an after-dinner stroll with my wife and son on the University of North Carolina campus by passing out. We were visitors this Labor Day weekend to the USA Baseball National Training Complex in nearby Cary. My son was selected to join other thirteen-year-old baseball players from New England for a few days of humility at the hands of teams from California, Georgia, Texas, and other hothouses of baseball talent. The beating from the sun was equally relentless that day. Later, my head lost a scuffle with the sidewalk, as heads often do.

I also aspirated souvlaki with yogurt dressing into my lungs. Oxygen had to compete with my partially digested dinner. "A Mediterranean diet is healthy as long as you keep it out of your lungs," I whispered to my doctor, my voice raspy, my chest burning with each inhalation. I forced a few deep breaths hoping the oxygen level would rise. The monitor wanted nothing to do with my parlor tricks.

Another large IV. More blood samples. A second EKG. Chest X-ray—"take a deep breath and hold." Sitting up on the ER gurney—breathing was easier—I found myself the object of attention and the subject of an experience. I was a citizen health-care provider, fluent in the language. I understood the patois pocked with abbreviations—low pulse ox, ST elevations—and terms like hypoxia, tachycardia, and soft blood pressure spoken around me. And yet, at that moment, the entire situation felt strange and otherworldly. I thought, "How can any patient not feel intimidated and lost in this space?"

My perspective shift could be explained by my unexpected position, the result of wearing an uncomfortable gown and not a stethoscope. But it also diminishes my experience by slotting it into a category with other stories where the doctor finds insight after being a patient. My story becomes a type of story, and in doing so, ceases to be mine.

I have a healthy suspicion for neat narratives, the cozy moral. Life is messy and difficult to penetrate. In medicine, there's a tendency to force experiences into a script or into a diagnosis. I'm not saying such gestures are wrong or untrue; they're just inauthentic in certain situations.

Even as I write these words, I struggle to fully understand how we come to describe and understand our experiences. In "The Poetics of Space," Gaston Bachelard writes, "We must look for centers of simplicity in homes with many rooms. . . . In a palace, 'there's no place for intimacy.'" Hospital ERs, spaces with rooms upon rooms, designed with more empathy for technology than humans, risk leaving patients feeling like uninvited but tolerated guests. The challenge becomes taking these spaces and creating simplicity and intimacy that coexist with monitors, fear, and patients' complicated narratives.

I wasn't the medical trainwreck suggested by my medical history, though I recognized my problems were difficult to ignore. Open-heart surgery. Mitral valve repair. Atrial fibrillation. Multiple cardiac ablations. A period of rate-related cardiomyopathy that weakened the heart muscle. For a time, I was on the same medications as my heart failure patients. And yet, recovery put that turmoil in the past. With denial's expert help, I considered myself healthy.

Luckily, my wife contacted the on-call physician for my internist, who had access to previous EKGs. The concerning changes in my EKG were old, a remnant of prior injury and surgery. My doctors sighed in relief. My response was more somber. I could ignore my past struggles, pretend they no longer matter, but indelible tracings remain. The body betrays as much as it conceals.

Syncope is the medical term for a transient loss of consciousness with spontaneous recovery resulting from inadequate blood flow to the brain. Interestingly, another meaning for syncope is to contract a word by omitting middle sounds or letters. When you pass out, you become cut off from your experience and the return feels like an unwrinkling of the senses. Voices floated in my head, then entered my ears as strange faces emerged into tighter focus. "Dude, you passed out," a slurred voice said, standing over me, holding a red solo cup. It was the opening home game for the University of North Carolina football team, and there were parties everywhere.

"Dude. You have a few?"

I tried to tell him I hadn't been drinking, but he kept asking. I can only assume people were partying hard and hitting the ground harder on this beautiful and festive evening. His brain made assumptions and created a believable story. It was easier to marvel at my condition than to be curious about it.

The sound of my son's voice settled me. "You okay? Don't touch your head, Dad. You're bleeding." He was half-naked, pressing his T-shirt to my bleeding scalp, terrified.

Once in the back of the ambulance, lying on the gurney, I felt the doors slam closed more than I heard them. I saw

my wife frantically talking to the medics, who were pointing and directing her to the hospital. The sunlight had softened into nightfall when EMS started the engine. Red lights
strobed through the street, dispersing onlookers. I followed
my wife and son, running to our car, their bodies growing
smaller as we pulled away, thinking, "I'm not making it to
the hospital, I'll never see my family again."

This emotional run-in with my mortality had happened
only once, the day before my heart surgery. Then, I met it
by peddling the exercise bike. This time, I sank into the gurney and closed my eyes. There was a foreboding symmetry
to this disorientating experience, for it was Labor Day, ten
years earlier, when I nearly passed out while working in the
ER. I convinced colleagues that I was fine. The next day I was
admitted to the hospital with rapid atrial fibrillation and
pneumonia. The day after that, they diagnosed my lousy
heart valve. I started accumulating medical problems like
cheap coins, and my journey as a doctor–patient began.

"Stay with us," the medic said. I didn't like his tone,
reassurance with a vibrato of contained panic. He told me
he was starting an IV in my arm. I worried that the large-
gauge needle didn't hurt, that I was calm even though I
couldn't breathe. I heard the medics discuss my case over
the radio—my EKG, low oxygen level, and soft blood pressure. That's a worrisome story, I thought, bathing in sweat.

I was thinking on that moment later in the ER, after my
doctors and nurses left me alone, and the medics rolled in
a guy whose heart wasn't beating at all. I heard the familiar
orders of the code through the curtain separating us—the

call and response. I tried hard not to imagine my naked body on the stretcher getting cardiopulmonary resuscitation (CPR) and having a breathing tube pushed down my throat into my airway. I wondered what went through his mind when his heart stopped. Did he sense he was about to die? Was he convincing himself the discomfort was only indigestion? Was death a welcome relief from pain and dependency or a source of sudden fear? These questions became a matter of surprising urgency. I could tell from their tone the doctors didn't expect this resuscitation to be successful. It wasn't long before the time of death was called, the team dispersed, and the poor guy was left alone, just as I've done after codes throughout my career.

I peeked through the gaps in the portable curtains. The nurses wrapped the body in a white sheet. A life, however, can't be bundled that easily. They wheeled his body away. I hoped he was off to a viewing room filled with teary-eyed family and friends. His doctors, I knew too well, weren't thinking about the man anymore. They were busy with the bureaucracy of death. Talk to any family. Fill out the death certificate. Call the medical examiner and the organ bank. Having no responsibility for him, I had the luxury to mull over the life left behind.

My wife came into the room, her worry taking on a different type of pale. "That's the first time I've ever seen a dead person," she said.

In that moment, I thought back to my ambulance ride, the belief that I wasn't going to make it to the hospital. What if I was the code called overhead? What if I was the first dead person my wife and son ever saw? Thinking on certain possibilities produced a pain so unlike anything else that it's easier not to consider it. What's in the "it"? Fear of dying? The distress of leaving the people I love so much? I'm still rummaging through the "it."

There's an unfathomable gravity to the ER space, where lives in crisis pass through and some depart forever. We can't forget the word "patient" is derived from the Latin *patiens*, which means "to suffer." Whether it's failing bodies, bad choices, the fear of losing control, or morphing identities, suffering is a deeply personal matter. Sometimes, it's the story that runs beneath or in between the stories being told, undetected by beeping monitors.

The embarrassment was unbearable. I had passed out in front of my son. I was bloodied and covered in vomit. A father wants to display strength to his son. That's hard when you can't even compete against gravity. I was told he was terrified when I hit the ground. Apparently, I jerked a little, too. Probably myoclonic jerks. Intellectualizing the experience is easier than imagining what my son was feeling, especially when I passed out just when my wife left him to look out for me as she ran for the car.

An ER patient should have time to ruminate on matters such as death and fear and embarrassment, but I discovered we get interrupted, too. EMS pushed a mouthy drunk driver into the newly emptied spot on the other side of the screen. "Keep your neck collar on," I heard a doctor or a nurse say, followed by mechanical words I've used so many times myself: "We're trying to help you."

ERs and hospitals are designed to be healing spaces, but people are the sources of intimacy and warmth. Stories open up to other stories once you try to tell it. I remember the jokes the CT techs told me as they moved me into the scanner, the concern from a former medical student now training in emergency medicine, afraid of violating privacy laws but she saw my name on the board, the nurse who swaddled me in blankets when I couldn't stop shivering throughout the night. I was discharged from the hospital the following morning to fly home, where I became sicker and then slowly recovered.

A story is a house with many rooms. Bringing order to any story is challenging. The present can't always shake memory's shadows or prevent thoughts about the future from echoing off the walls.

Before this incident in Chapel Hill, I spent a few years in atrial fibrillation, an irregularly irregular heart rhythm. I continued to run three to four miles most days of the week. My heart raced, and over time it became damaged and weakened from overwork, a condition called cardiomyopathy. Simple walking made me breathless. I collapsed on the couch when I came home from an ER shift. I needed a last-ditch ablation, and if it didn't hold, my cardiologist mumbled the word transplant. My body was the problem, but the deep hurt, I later realized, was the possibility of not being able to provide for my family, of being a reduced version of myself, and thus, becoming a different self altogether.

The cardiac ablation was a success. Electrophysiologists must first map the heart's aberrant electrical impulses, a feat as astonishing and inscrutable as a city power grid. Then they zap these intruders, erecting a line of defense so my sinus node, the heart's steady pacemaker, can do its work uninterrupted. Some experiences are harder to map. I've rewritten this piece countless times. I can't describe the scene in the ambulance, pulling away from my wife and son, without tears filling my eyes. I was scared, aware that my medical knowledge couldn't protect me. We strive for strength and resilience, but to get there we must sometimes tip a respectful nod to vulnerability and frailty.

Around five years after passing out, I was invited to give a late-afternoon talk at a Midwest medical school where the newly installed emergency medicine chair was none other than the ER attending who supervised my care that evening in Chapel Hill. We shook hands and exchanged pleasantries. After a few minutes, I realized he didn't remember caring for me. I jogged his memory, but I was convinced his acknowledgment was nothing more than politeness. I felt slighted, then happy. You don't want to be the patient everyone remembers. When intense experiences populate a typical ER shift, the background blurs, making it hard for a singular experience to stand out. Luckily, my notable experience was, for him, just another case.

11
Waiting for the Surge

You track the wave of cases. It's April 2020, and there are over 10,000 COVID-19 deaths in New York City alone as cases mount in Boston. Models predict that Rhode Island, your state, your community, and your hospital will be overrun in a week or two. For now, you're waiting for the surge.

During your last ER shift, almost all your patients were infected, or thought to be infected, with the virus that causes COVID-19. You can't distance yourself from the virus, but you need to keep your anxiety at arm's length. One strategy you improvise is the second-person point of view. "You" provides a six-feet separation to fragile emotional spaces. "You" gives you space to hear yourself while speaking directly to others; it's a personal and a community voice.

Friends you haven't heard from in years reach out. "How are you? Do you all have enough personal protective equipment?" People with contacts. Business associates, friends, cousins. So many cousins with connections. You love the way terms like PPE and R0 float off their tongues. Teachers, artists, writers, academics, business owners, all sound more informed and reasoned than governmental "experts" in pandemic response.

During an ER shift, one of your favorite nurses asks, "How are you?" You grin painfully. "I'm okay," you answer, and make a lame joke like you were never okay in the first place. "How about you?" She nods and says, "People say they're okay. But they're not okay."

Waiting for the surge, you sense what people are really feeling. They're scared. They're tired. They're figuring out whether there's a right amount of being scared and tired or is everyone on their own. It's a different type of fear. It's the terror that belongs to children who believe a monster is living in their closet and closing their eyes will make it appear.

You pretend you aren't bringing COVID-19 home with you from work. You remove your scrubs outside and pad downstairs to the washing machine in the basement. You're sure the neighbors see more of you than anyone should. Waiting for the surge, you fear their young children will be permanently scarred by this hairy man hopping around the other side of the fence.

Waiting for the surge, you pray for your family because they've been at home, strict practitioners of social distancing, and if they become infected it's all on you. Family discussions turn from summer plans to advance directives. You notice your son complains less about the changing face of his first year in college when the conversation turns to family finances, and all that he needs to do should his father become ill.

More COVID-19 patients fill your hospital. Waves of them from homeless shelters and nursing homes and multigenerational families who live closely together. The death toll rises.

You learn that breathing for eight hours—roughly 9,000 breaths—against the tight seal of an N95 mask is serious work. Your mouth turns dry. Your brain fogs like your goggles. You become dehydrated quickly, but when leaving the unit requires doffing your protective gear to pee, and then putting on fresh equipment, drinking fluids is now something you do sparingly.

Waiting for the surge, you can't sleep. Mindfulness fails. Any headspace you create fills with thoughts about all the deaths. Everyone is either fighting the surge or waiting for it to come. Pressure builds behind your watery eyes. Maybe it's your seasonal allergies, you tell yourself. Spring is pushing flowers from the ground. And despite repeated failures by government, there's compassion blooming all around, from people donating personal protective equipment to sewing masks at home, keeping each other fed, and soliciting gently used iPads so patients in hospitals can stay connected to their families. The only way out of this is through a shared purpose and a collective voice.

You wait for the surge through a mutual point of view. "You" doesn't let us forget that individual exposure risk is tied to societal behavior, that we're responsible and accountable for each other. "You" can be an insistent and urgent voice.

The surge is upon you now. As you walk the neighborhood after a shift, a neighbor driving by stops and rolls down his car window. "You're my hero," he says. "We wish you the best." You stand in the road awkwardly, chilled from the waning sunlight and the gusting winds. You're embarrassed. You're not a hero. You're an ER doc. Besides, the pandemic has produced so many heroes in hospitals and in communities. But the feeling behind his words breaks through the distance. I graciously accept his good wishes and stuff them deep into my pants pocket, thank him, and tell him to stay safe.

12
Narrative Risks: Shape, Place, and Gutter

The story of Carlos E doesn't grab the reader like many others from the frontlines of the COVID-19 pandemic. He isn't gasping for each breath, begging me not to let him die. He's not even an example of "happy hypoxia," a logic-defying phenomenon unique to COVID-19 where the oxygen level in a patient's bloodstream is low but they appear alarmingly comfortable. Carlos is a polite, gracious man in his early thirties, dressed in a crisp T-shirt, narrow cut jeans, and spotless white running shoes, with normal vital signs, a constellation of symptoms, and a desire to go to work and care for his young family. There's little obvious drama to this scene, or his story, which makes it precarious.

I met Carlos E in our dedicated COVID unit in the ER. Beds permitting, patients known to have COVID-19 or deemed a PUI, a "person under investigation," with a history and symptoms suspicious for SARS-CoV-2 infection, are triaged to this warm zone. Carlos checked several of these boxes.

Recent contacts with people with known COVID-19?

He recently visited family in New York City, a pandemic hotspot at the time.

Fever?

He felt warm but never took his temperature.

Cough?

Poquito, he says, pinching his thumb and forefinger together.

Sore throat?

He swallows.

Perhaps.

His hand rubbed at his belly, communicating abdominal discomfort but not pain. Gastrointestinal complaints had recently joined the list of suspicions symptoms for COVID-19, and he reports nausea, vomiting, and a loose bowel movement since early in the day.

Carlos E didn't want to come to the ER. It was early in the first wave of the pandemic, and his boss forced him. COVID-19 cases were growing in Rhode Island, and the governor hadn't yet shut the state down. His boss refused to let him work in the restaurant without first being checked out. Because of the limited number of testing kits and sites, we were seeing patients in the ER for the sole purposes of testing.

We fought two anxieties working in the ER on the cusp of the first COVID-19 surge in March 2020. First, pay attention at all times to reduce any risk of infection. And don't screw up by thinking only about whether patients have, or don't have, COVID-19.

COVID's shadow followed me as I moved from patient to Purell to computer to Purell to patient to Purell to utility room to wash my hands to answer the phone to remember that I hadn't disinfected the phone when I came on shift. So complete was COVID-19's gravitational pull on my physical and mental effort, I feared closing myself off to the usual non-pandemic diseases and problems.

The diagnostic process is complex. I've learned not to force the process when it doesn't come easy and distrust it when it does. The mind, or my mind, is prone to biases, to take cognitive shortcuts. Because this process operates unconsciously, we're often unaware that our apparently sound decisions are faulty, our confidence in them unearned.

Premature closure, quickly homing in on a particular diagnosis before you've gathered all the relevant data, is a bias frequently blamed for cognitive errors in medicine. Unfortunately, it permeates our daily lives as well. I suspect too many ugly relationship moments start with cutting off the speaker mid-sentence because we believe we know what the other person is about to say, only to find ourselves in the desert of wrong. In medicine, a suggestion to overcome this tendency is to keep a broad differential diagnosis, to remain open to many possible explanations, not just one.

This sounds easy in retrospect but unusually difficult when you're in the moment. How we incorporate and interpret fragments of information in decision-making is an ongoing investigation for cognitive science researchers and people like me, clinicians curious about how and why we create and value specific stories. These stories, the foundation of our decision-making, are themselves the products of decisions.

We're making decisions before we think we're making decisions. Stories aren't just heard, they're constructed. Both tellers and listeners are involved in the story-manufacturing process. Both parties choose certain details to work with and not others. The listener isn't passive, but is actively piecing together fragments of information and arranging them in a particular sequence. At this stage, I find my thinking susceptible to another common bias, the availability bias. The availability bias describes the inclination to judge things as more likely if they immediately come to mind. At the start of the pandemic, COVID-19 was a fragment foremost on our minds.

Even if two clinicians choose similar pieces of information, each might interpret them differently. An element of subjectivity enters into what we believe to be science-using and evidence-based decisions. The imagination can lead us astray, but it can also transport us beyond what's evident to what's missing, beyond what "is" to what "might be."

In a 1944 social psychology study, researchers Fritz Heider and Marianne Simmel showed subjects a simple animated movie where a large triangle, a small triangle, and a circle moved in various directions and at various speeds about a screen. Then, they asked research subjects to describe what they saw. Respondents took these inanimate shapes that lacked any innate personality, personal history, or motivation, and described drama, bullying, jealousy, and romance. Only one person described what their eyes observed—moving geometric objects.

When I played this film for students, they took this ambiguous visual information and created confident, specific, and even passionate narratives. A lesbian love story with the disapproving father—big triangle—leaving the two woman no choice but to run away together. Someone else described the big triangle as angry and the smaller triangle and circle as friendly, which further upset the big triangle. In yet another interpretation, the circle is unfaithful to the big triangle. People saw a terrified mother and child escaping from an abusive father, a war between shapes causing destruction, children at recess, jealousy and love, males and females, aggressors and victims.

In emergency medicine, how we frame the story dictates which details to prioritize. That Carlos E doesn't want to be here tinted how I weigh the other details in his story. The sole purpose of the visit was work clearance. He shouldn't have to come to the ER for a COVID-19 test and potentially become exposed to the virus in our unit. Why weren't there enough tests, anyway? These unrelated system frustrations about the national response filtered into my encounter with Carlos E, who, like many patients, won't be happy when he learns he'll need to self-quarantine at home and miss work until his test comes back in a few days.

At the beginning of the pandemic, we compared how and to what degree positive cases resembled one another or presented differently. Understanding patients in this relational manner is typical in medicine. Experienced clinicians draw on a bank of tens of thousands of encounters over the expanse of their careers to inform their impression of a single case. However, we don't typically examine how our impression of each patient's story is influenced by its relation to and association with people and cases in immediate proximity to it.

This phenomenon deserves attention in clinical practice because it's been skillfully employed to manipulate and engage moviegoers dating back to the 1920s. At that time, film was a new medium, and Lev Kuleshov, a Russian filmmaker and one of the first film theorists, made a film that interspersed an actor's face between images of a woman, a bowl of soup, and a corpse. Audiences praised the actor's imperceptible expression of lust, hunger, and grief. But when the actor's expression is examined closely, it was the same face, the same exact expression. Their interpretation was informed by the images associated with it. Kuleshov wrote that art depends on two attributes, the material itself and how the artist organizes the material. Film editing can create an impression of a coherent narrative even from a seemingly disconnected series of images.

An ER shift can feel like managing an endless montage of experiences where I serve as an editor shaping perception and the recipient influenced by this unconscious manipulation. Everyday, Kuleshov's insights from a hundred years ago influence my interpretation of what might be going on with patients. In the warm zone during the COVID-19 pandemic, the narrative energy was directed around the question of COVID-19.

The results of Carlos E's blood work trickle in. The labs and chest X-ray are reassuring. Perfect oxygen level. Many patients in that warm unit followed that paradigm. Carlos E wanted to go home. I wanted to get him home. I rehearse in my head the conversation I would repeat hundreds of times: self-isolation, facial coverings, take your temperature until the COVID-19 test results in a few days.

Cough, sore throat, nausea, vomiting, diarrhea, abdominal pain, recent visit to New York City. These details fit the image of COVID-19. I made it fit. Because they fit so well, I wasn't aware of the connections I'd made, the spaces between fragments that are as important as the fragments themselves.

The power of these in-between spaces is evident to anyone who has read comics, which I suspect is most of us. They're called gutters. Scott McLoud describes gutters in his book *Making Comics* as the empty spaces between comic panels where readers make connections and weave disjointed visual sequences into a coherent narrative.

Scott McCloud shows us a panel where a character wields an ax. Screams follow in the next panel. One concludes the attacker hurt if not killed someone. But we don't know. Maybe the presumed victim fought back, or the attacker slipped or was felled by a back spasm brought on by raising that heavy ax. You get the point. As readers, we instinctively and actively make assumptions. The graphic artist counts on us to fill in the gaps, to play with our expectations and generate tension. Comics function as low tech and often brilliant instruments that illuminate the imaginative leaps we take when caring for patients, where the gutters are not well marked and the narrative frames less explicit.

During a typical ER shift, one is bombarded with new patients, information from patients, family, health providers and consultants, and diagnostic testing. Efficiency demands that we constantly sort and edit this sensory and cognitive load of oral, visual, and written material. Our brain's craving for narrative coherence is part of decision-making. Daniel Kahneman writes how our mind is predisposed to jump to conclusions, to take information that's available and make a story. It neglects ambiguity and is impatient with doubt. It doesn't bother with details it doesn't have. If we don't recognize these cognitive shortcuts, we're in danger of creating an easier story or a more convenient story, which might differ from the story the patient is telling.

I found myself moving quickly with Carlos E's care. At the time, the question was straightforward. Do I suspect he has COVID-19 and is he well enough to be discharged?

While typing the medical decision-making portion of Carlos E's chart—an effort of intentional inefficiency since I think differently punching keys than dictating—his story became objectified on the screen, and the pieces connected differently in my head. Carlos E had a slight fever, another finding that's consistent with a COVID-19 diagnosis. But his abdomen pain was still there, vague and gnawing. He tells me it's nothing. But his belly was tender in the right lower quadrant where the appendix lives. Fever, nausea, vomiting, loose stools, abdominal pain. His symptoms were so classic for appendicitis that a third-year medical student could have nailed it. The CT scan showed a thickened appendix with surrounding inflammation. He could have both, of course. Appendicitis and COVID-19. But he didn't.

We rarely question story validity the way we do research validity. Research studies must follow rigorous research methods and use sound statistical analysis. And yet, we don't subject stories to similar scrutiny. We must be vigilant of story's charms. The elements that account for a story's power and imaginative force may also lead the unwitting listener astray.

13
Zebras

The hospital gown lies on the floor at the foot of the ER stretcher.

The police found Sally B resting in a small cemetery beside a local church in a New England city that peaked during the Industrial Revolution. She pushed herself up and walked with them to the police car when they asked her, though she thought it a crazy idea. She's a zebra, and there's no way a zebra is going to fit into the back seat of a police car.

"We expect all patients to change into a gown," I say.

She's lounging on the ER stretcher on her side, propped on her elbow, hand hidden behind frizzed brambles of auburn hair.

"I can't," she says, her lips spotted with lipstick, her smile warm with pity.

She looks smart in blue jeans and a white T-shift stretched at the neck. Swollen ankles overwhelm her expensive-looking brown penny loafers.

"I'll step out and give you some privacy."

Her eyelids flutter with profound disbelief. "Thank you. But I can't. You know I can't."

"I don't understand," I say, unable to hide my confusion.

Her face explodes with disbelief. "Are you really a doctor?"

"I am."

"Wow," she says, amazed, shaking her head with such conviction I wonder whether she's privy to something lacking in me that I must be concerned about. She looks around the curtained space, takes it all in, and sighs. "I'm a zebra."

"I heard. But we still need you to change into a gown."

"C'mon," she says, now with a sparkle to her eye. "You'll see my stripes."

14
Hug, or Ugh

Fawn was bouncing on the edge of her stretcher, a homeless woman in her late fifties, feet drumming on the scuffed tiles like that of an impatient schoolgirl. She was hurling insults at EMS when they rolled her into the ER. They had found her asleep outside the police station. The triage nurse knew her from previous visits—mental health problems and substance use, cocaine mostly, sometimes heroin. I extended my hand and introduced myself.

When I stepped into the exam room, she popped upright. "Hi, doctor," she said, grabbing my hand. Without letting go, before I could even say another word, she looked up at me with desperate, bloodshot eyes and asked for a hug.

"A hug?" I said.

"Yes, doctor," she said. She ranted about living in shelters, and how, sure, she'd made mistakes in her life, but don't believe the EMS bullshit about drugs; maybe a little crack and a nip here and there, but she's no addict, and what can she do when she has nobody, nobody in the world to prove them wrong. "Just a hug?" she begged.

The weight of each passing second counted against me as I took in her sun-roughened face, the wrinkles scuffed with dirt, and her dirty jeans and oversized T-shirt. The air around her smelled of someone going through a tough time—old sweat, stale cigarettes, and greasy food. In my emergency medicine education, I was trained to respond quickly to a wide variety of urgent situations. At no time did I come across one that was urgent in this way. My muscles tensed. My heart cramped.

I opened my arms.

We hugged.

To be completely honest, she hugged me. She pressed the side of her head against my chest. The weave of my heavy white coat suddenly porous and inadequate between us the longer she stayed there. I politely nudged her off.

"Okay," I said, gently coaxing her away. Only with a little forceful encouragement did she return to her seat on the stretcher. "What's going on?" I asked.

Stories raced from her mouth, a runaway thought-train: bogus arrests, undeserved jail time, bad marriages, field hockey and soccer stardom back in high school, ungrateful children, hospitalizations for being "bipolar," no sleep for five days straight—no, six.

She appeared comfortable with me. No longer yelling, she returned to the stretcher. But an uneasiness swept down my body. I found myself disengaged from the scene as the words cascaded off her chapped lips. Did I just hug this patient? I thought. My chest was itching now. People playing out the formality of a hug often lean forward at the shoulders without committing the chest. The casual hug is often shoulder-to-shoulder, a buddy hug. Fawn pressed the side of her head firmly against my sternum.

The hug left an invisible imprint that remained long after we separated. I couldn't decide whether it was the hug itself or a hug with her.

Shortly after, back at the computer, I casually informed a senior emergency medicine resident about Fawn's request for a hug. The resident chuckled. "Yeah. She asked me for a hug, too."

"Oh," I said. Nothing particularly agreeable about me, such as my demeanor or nonverbal communication skills, prompted the request. She was asking everyone. "What did you do?" I asked.

She scoffed, as if the answer was obvious. "I told her there were professional boundaries."

"Sure," I said. That was a nice way of wording it. I kicked myself for not thinking of that. But boundary violations in the doctor–patient relationship typically center on sexual misconduct and behavior that exploits a patient's vulnerability. Fawn made an explicit request for a hug.

I'm not necessarily obligated to comply with a patient's every wish. Suppose a patient asks for antibiotics to treat a viral infection. In that case, I may suggest other methods of treatment because antibiotics won't work and the requested therapy carries potential risks, such as a drug allergy, interactions with other drugs on the patient's med list, or potential

Clostridium difficile colitis. Under the hood of any medical decision, I'm balancing benefits and risks for the patient, not the interests of the doctor.

A hug, I realize, isn't needless antibiotics; it's more complicated than that, and perhaps the medical treatment paradigm doesn't apply here. As a physical display, it appears straightforward, but it's as primal, emotionally rich, and perilous as any poem. There are subtle variables—from the placement of hands, the position of the body, and the pressure exerted—that can alter the meaning of the hug. The context matters, too. A light hug between acquaintances is not the same as a hug between relatives or the hug shared by mourners or the hug during a first date.

To initiate a hug is an exercise in extreme vulnerability. By opening the arms, the hugger exposes themselves to rejection. There's always a risk of being turned down, of not being accepted. A hug isn't a promise, it's a question. With Fawn, there was no middle ground. Refusing a hug at that moment seemed as inexcusable and avoidable as any other form of hospital-related harm.

I confessed to a few ER staff what I'd done.

"Don't touch your wife when you get home," said one nurse.

"Shower and boil your clothes very first thing," said someone else.

They squirmed as if I'd just dropped a Swedish fish candy onto the hospital floor and eaten it. Yes, there are situations where the five-second-rule does not apply. I was now unsure whether the hug counted as an admirable or a regrettable act.

These young doctors and seasoned nurses were more than superb clinicians, they were the embodiment of kindness and sensitivity. And yet, I was stunned to see my hug greeted with disbelief and a touch of horror. Maybe my dress complicated matters. At the time, before the COVID-19 pandemic, I wore regular street clothes when working in the ED, not scrubs. This commingling of my personal life and professional role as an ER doc might have muddled their perception and heightened their visceral response. What part and how much of me was involved in that hug? If I was walking on the street and Fawn asked for a hug, would I acquiesce? I know the answer I'd like to give.

"Doctor? Hey, doctor!"

Fawn kept calling for me over the next few hours. She wasn't done talking. I popped into her exam room but ventured only as far as the doorway. She rambled on about the problems she'd already told me. I nodded, repeated the plans for the social worker and the psychiatrist to talk with her, and found ways to extract myself. Soon, I took detours when my path to other patients' rooms pulled me across her line of sight. She started bothering the unit clerk sitting at the desk across from her room. "The doctor's busy," I overhead, again and again.

I reconsidered the hug. Was it a blameworthy act? Did it signify something about me or our relationship that wasn't intended? Had I returned the hug in a manner that conveyed unvoiced pledges of larger commitments? I did smile afterward. Maybe she misread my politeness?

Fawn's workup didn't raise any acute medical problems that required immediate attention, and we waited on psychiatry to evaluate her mania and disorganized thinking.

At home that evening, my own reasoning about her remained disorganized. Professional boundaries provided a justifiable intellectual explanation for dodging a hug, but felt thin and emotionally dishonest. The professional boundaries argument in Fawn's case cloaked unspoken biases about her, her lifestyle, her aesthetic; mental and social problems beyond our reach, and if her past proved prescient, beyond hers as well.

I washed my clothes, scrubbed myself in the shower. And yet, a maddening discomfort remained on my skin. It wasn't the lingering residue of physical contact but the realization that the hug itself was a lie.

I'm not an indiscriminate hugger. Research shows that people with traits of extroversion such as sociability and spontaneity are your prototypical huggers, while those who are more anxious, who suffer from a lack of self-confidence and self-esteem, like me, are not. But I hug. I reserve hugs and other gestures of embrace for people I hold with great affection. But I don't carry this policy with strict consistency, either. I've hugged in the ER before. There are little kids and sweet grandmothers who have made my day with a hug. They were strangers to me before they came to the ER, and yet I've glowed from these gestures of intimacy for the very reason that these strangers were moved to do so. The hug was an expression of gratitude, a statement of true emotional connection. Such moments highlight any ER clinician's shift, necessary reminders about why I practice medicine. In these moments, hugs are celebrations of melting boundaries, not violations of tender physical and emotional territories.

Part of the problem is that Fawn hugged quickly—too quickly. I sensed that my position as the physician supervising her care didn't matter. I stood as a surrogate for the absent people in her life, those she needed who had abandoned or even wronged her. And maybe I hugged her for dubious reasons, too. The gesture concealed my unacknowledged biases and the fact I could do little to improve the circumstances of her life. However, a hug might epitomize the most cost-effective magic bullet I could offer.

An argument can be made that a hug deserves recognition as a bona fide medical treatment. It harbors positive biochemical and physiological benefits, associated with lower blood pressure, stress reduction, stabilizing mood, and forging trust. A hug can raise the level of oxytocin, the "love hormone" that promotes mother–infant bonding and serves a role in altruistic giving. In the United States and other countries, there's a National Hugging Day, created on the premise that consensual hugging improves physical, emotional, and spiritual health. Even so, the hug is not without risks.

This incident took place well over a decade ago.

Would I hug Fawn today? In the era of #MeToo, I'm much more alert to any gesture that others, especially patients, might misinterpret. Touch is a powerful communication tool. Individuals who observe tactile behavior can detect, with various degrees of accuracy, emotions such as anger, fear, disgust, love, and sympathy without experiencing the stimulation firsthand. But the ability to "read" or appreciate the meaning of a hug relies on many factors beyond our control. A hug is informed by the background, the personality, the motivation, and the culture of the people involved. Unwanted touching, under the rule of law, is battery.

But what about necessary touching? During the COVID-19 pandemic, I felt a growing need for touch from patients, especially those who were older. They were alone, cared for by doctors, nurses, and ER techs shielded behind face masks, gowns, and layers of gloves. Once infectious risk and inadequate personal protection became a dominant storyline, simple touch and proximity began to resemble other medical interventions, subject to scrutiny of benefits and risks. Fearing what was lost by minimizing touch, the symbolic expression of warm concern, I took to stating the obvious to patients: "We're going to take good care of you." After this remark, I noticed their tendency to reach for my hand and squeeze. Unlike the pre-COVID-19 handshakes, these handshakes had the force of Fawn's hug, as if needing reassurance that a human heart was beating behind all the protection.

Fawn is a fiftyish-year-old woman with a history of mental illness, polysubstance use, and homelessness, who presents to the ER by EMS acting agitated after being found on the sidewalk. This opening line will foreground her case presentation. But it misses critical pieces of her story. The slight tremors I detected in her face as she waited for my response. Her need for a hug and the tension I experienced complying with her request. Was my hug a genuine connection, or was it no different from the sizzling crack high she was addicted to, a short-lived reward that left her craving more? In the end, I fear the hug was a morally suspect gesture. I wasn't hugging her. I was hugging her loneliness, a life spinning out of control. Maybe she wasn't hugging me either, but seeking momentary stability, someone or something to hold onto.

II
Constraints

The task of a writer is not to solve the problem but to state the problem correctly.

—Anton Chekhov

15
Moving On

Kevin A, barely twenty, lies bloody and broken on a gurney in the emergency department. He was ejected through the front windshield of his friend's car as it rammed into a telephone pole. It's hard to look at his bruised face, swollen beyond his eyes, and bloody mouth without feeling as if my own teeth are breaking into pieces.

During the ambulance ride, his thready pulse vanished, though the medics admitted they weren't sure he ever had one, couldn't say whether what they felt was a sign of life or something they willed onto the young man. Regardless, Kevin's heart isn't beating now. The trauma team cracks open his rib cage and sternum in search of blood filling the sac around the heart, or a hemorrhage from one of the large blood vessels running through the chest. This procedure, called a thoracotomy, is always a last-ditch effort and rarely works.

As the time of death is called, the silence descending over the trauma room is shattered by angry yells from the driver of the car. He's in a trauma room across the hall, intoxicated, screaming at the staff, and ignorant to the tragic fates of his passenger-friends. The back-seat passenger is in another trauma room. She will survive, but owing to her injuries she will probably lead a life very different from the one of unbridled promise she possessed earlier that evening.

The team in Kevin's room—doctors and nurses, techs and social workers—conceal their feelings of sadness, grief, injustice, and rage. We share looks without actually looking at one another.

There's so much to absorb and process. The senseless death of a young man we had no chance of saving; the irresponsible drunk driver now causing a ruckus. Yet we don't talk about it. Instead, we disperse and seek safe harbor in our respective duties and rituals. We document. We clean the body. We notify the organ bank. We rip off blood-streaked gowns and gloves and toss them into garbage bins. We snap a fresh sheet over Kevin's body and brace for the families to arrive.

And we move on.

"That's what we do," the senior emergency medicine resident said to me the following night at the hospital for another overnight shift. I'd confessed how the case had followed me home when I got off my shift. The resident admitted that he hadn't slept well either. A nurse described being similarly haunted.

"But that's what we do, right? Move on?" the resident said.

I nodded. The nurse nodded. But what did we agree to with those ready nods? I don't believe we were attesting to the factual accuracy of this statement, but acknowledging an unspoken truth. Our relationship to tragedy is inadequate, even warped, and yet we never take the time to talk about it.

How can any caring human being move on after being face-to-face with a human heart that a short time ago pumped with life and promise? But moving on is embedded into emergency medicine practice. Simultaneously juggling the sick, the not so sick, and the needy. Handling a mix of complex patient workups, procedures, and conversations. When there's too much to do and too little time, focusing on any one activity means falling behind in others. We move on because desperation and efficiency demand that we do so. We move on because it's often an easy and justifiable excuse for not dealing with our emotions. What makes our work difficult can be very different from what makes it profoundly hard.

When physicians suffer, patients may suffer, too. When my emotional reserve drops, it means I have a limited supply of what my patients deserve—compassion, patience, and a willingness to follow unwinding stories. Despite attempts at bravura, emergency medicine clinicians, along with other frontline specialists, smolder with precarious rates of depression and burnout. Burnout is a syndrome marked by depersonalization, emotional exhaustion, and a low sense of personal accomplishment. I respect this thing called burnout while remaining skeptical of any categorizing scheme that tries to squeeze a heterogeneous set of factors into one package.

Many influences contribute to burnout in medicine. They include lack of control over the work environment, a disparity between personal values and those of the system, more time spent with electronic health records than with patients, and a sense of not making a difference. The medical-legal climate adds heat to this pot. There are stressors specific to emergency medicine that place its practitioners at further risk for burnout, including shift work and the constant exposure to patients suffering from extreme physical and emotional trauma. These systemic challenges serve as potent and poignant ingredients to burnout, but they measure out and interact and cook up differently for each physician. Thinking about it as a unified entity depersonalizes an individual's experience, which I fear may contribute to feelings of burnout.

The "it's what we do" mental trap is depersonalization in action. This attitude is a fascinating construction. The face of diligence and duty distances and distracts us from that which is painful and often terrifying. It gives us permission to look away and provides a ready defense to justify it. Moving on might be what we do, but that doesn't make it right or healthy.

I was introduced to "it's what we do" long before I was a physician. I was a sophomore in college in the early 1980s, volunteering at a local hospital ER over winter break, when I witnessed my first patient in cardiac arrest. This community hospital was a box off a suburban turnpike. The ER was a single space with a handful of beds separated by curtains. The small staff of nurses and ER techs threw themselves on this nursing home patient. Intubation, CPR, IV lines. I watched the staff, the medics, the doctor, and tried not to look at the body—the bald head and blank eyes, the pasty, cadaver-like toes shaking with each chest compression. I hardened my face, gulped down the sour sickening my stomach. Before long, the doctor called the time of death and returned to his morning coffee and bagel. And I went back to folding sheets and towels in the supply closet.

My unexpressed reactions to that experience broke through later that night while watching a rerun of the comedy *The Odd Couple*. I was sitting in the den of my parents' house, laughing at Oscar and Felix one minute, bawling the next. It came out of nowhere but from a definite somewhere. Maybe laughter softened the protective wall I'd erected and grief took advantage of that vulnerability. I felt a wave of sorrow for this man I never knew and mourned the life that no longer was. Until that morning, death was a devastating event. It produced shock. It ripped people apart. Never had I regarded death as an inconvenience, a disruption to one's breakfast. This was before the television series *ER*, before all the ER "reality" shows. To the uninitiated, the act of saving this fragile, older man looked like an assault. I was volunteering in this ER because I had become fascinated with medicine and felt inspired to go to medical school. At this moment, I saw inside the romantic idea of saving a life. A dread of what I might become grew alongside my dreams of medical school and what I wished to be.

None of the ER staff pulled me aside and asked how I was doing that morning. Decades later, I work in the ER of a busy teaching hospital, and I confess I'm not always sensitive to the shadowing medical student witnessing their first code. I miss opportunities to check in with them. Once, during an overnight shift, an eager medical student took over cardiac compressions during a code. He asked about the crunching sound in the chest. Broken ribs, we said. Terror gripped his face. Sometimes we break ribs, we said. I watched this gruesome reality wash over him. I feared he'd pass out, another cold reminder of all that's profound and devastating but rendered commonplace in the ER.

Sadly, the death of a Kevin A, a young man, is a familiar story, another entry in the ledger of senseless deaths and tragedies that make up the ambient reality of work in a trauma center. Whether moving on is the product of this dulled resignation or the root of the problem, I can't say. Regardless, Kevin's death hit me in a vulnerable place. That a young man's heart lay exposed and unprotected before me and I didn't feel a chill is a reason to shiver.

So did imagining tomorrow for the driver of the crash who, once he woke up, would face a life-long hangover of sadness and regret. The "it's what we do" ethos protected me from admitting what I was thinking about him at that very moment: the capricious and cruel manner in which fate doles out suffering to some people and spares others.

Kevin's untimely and unspeakable death tested the limits of this impulse to move on, and the purpose and pride we invest in it. Eventually, it exacts a cost. A numb heart is hard to recognize until it begins to warm and nerve endings crackle to life. When it hurts, it's a pain of longing, a reckoning. We ask ourselves how we felt nothing before and what else have I not been feeling that will disturb me later?

When the shell of "it's what we do" cracked open, it bared Kevin's death, the mechanical and often brutish things we do to bodies in a trauma code, the many lives irrevocably changed by the crash. These chilling experiences need to be felt, not blindly endured.

I tell the emergency medicine resident and nurse that I screwed up. I should have brought the team together for a few minutes after we pronounced Kevin dead. Trauma centers have described "the pause," a moment of silence after an unsuccessful resuscitation. It gives all of us around the stretcher the time and permission to honor the life that once was and to feel the gravity of the moment. These opportunities of respectful silence are now common in pockets of ERs around the country, including ours. If family members were in the resuscitation room watching the code, you hear their tears if you hadn't before. Unable to move on, we're forced to feel the air pressure change, recognize our proximity to the fragility of life, how it can make our work hard as well as a privilege.

I believe Kevin's death deserved a complete stop, even if it meant locking the door so nobody could run away. Sure, everyone had urgent tasks to do, but most of them could wait. Such a break in the action would not only honor Kevin and the other lives altered by this tragedy, but remind us that such deaths are never normal, and we shouldn't pretend otherwise.

16
Compassion at the Crossroads

It's taken a while, but Mr. Green, a heavy drinker, is finally sober enough to be discharged from the emergency department. As I examine him, I note that his scuffed hands aren't shaking. His speech isn't slurred. His gait is steady and proud. When an EMS crew pushed Mr. Green into the ER seven hours earlier, the alcohol in his bloodstream was at a level that would send most social drinkers into a coma. The ER staff knows Mr. Green very well. He's been in the ER almost every day for the past week, twice in the past twenty-four hours, and too many times to count over the years. His body shakes with withdrawal at a blood alcohol level where most people are considered drunk. We've monitored him meticulously, striving for that sweet spot of intoxication where he's finally functioning as if sober. But he's a homeless man and the clock shows 1:35 a.m. and we have a problem. It's a problem that can't be solved without creating another one. And the root of it, sadly enough, is compassion.

As I help him up by the elbow, I'm reminded how my feet slid on the icy pavement and the wind numbed my checks when I rushed from the parking lot into the hospital to start my shift. I blew warmth into cupped, stiff hands even after the ER doors shut behind me. Discharging Mr. Green means he will spend the night on the streets. Can I willfully send him outside, into the same brutal conditions I was so thankful to escape from? Providing compassionate care means letting him sleep until daylight when the shelter doors open.

Except the waiting room is filled, and every ER bed occupied. We are actively evaluating a few patients, but most patients have already been admitted into the hospital for many hours. They are boarding in the ER until beds open up in the hospital's wards and ICUs. The exodus of patients to hospital beds upstairs won't happen until late morning and early afternoon, so we need every possible ER bed to tend to those waiting to be seen and those who continue to arrive. The crisis of emergency department crowding turns the bed occupied by Mr. Green into a precious scarce resource. It also forces physicians like me to allocate compassion.

Crowding and prolonged waits in the ER are more than an inconvenience; they're linked to grave medical consequences, including higher inpatient mortality, longer length of stay in the hospital, increased medical errors, more harmful cardiac outcomes, and delayed treatment for pain. Moving patients from the waiting room to an ER bed as expediently as possible is the best strategy for timely and accurate treatment. The tired grandmother could be having a heart attack; the anxious entrepreneur could have a pulmonary embolus; the sleepy young man known for using drugs might have a brain infection.

On nights such as this one, triage nurses gather vital signs and prioritize patients with illness or injury that require immediate attention. The triage process isn't designed or staffed at night for deep dives into patient problems. Nurses must juggle the line of new patients at their window while appeasing those people who have been waiting for hours, many of whom are demonstrably and justifiably upset.

Letting Mr. Green sleep safe and warm sounds compassionate and comforting, but separating him from his alcohol puts him at risk for withdrawal. Sleeping too long can result in medical harm. If he were on the street, he'd "treat" himself by drinking again. I can stave off his alcohol withdrawal with benzodiazepines, a class of drugs used to treat anxiety and other problems. But a side effect of these medications is sedation, potentially delaying his discharge in the morning and taking up a bed even longer because now he's zonked out.

Mr. Green isn't seeking help for his alcoholism and homelessness. Our social workers and interdisciplinary care teams have tried to help him. He's been in and out of detox programs and burned so many bridges that they won't welcome him back even if they had beds. When in alcohol withdrawal, he has a habit of leaving the hospital AMA (against medical advice) shortly after being admitted.

Despite the countless turkey sandwiches and juices and warm, safe rooms to sleep, my care for Mr. Green never feels like care. Instead, I function as more of an accomplice, complicit in satisfying his short-term needs on his road to self-destruction.

It's easy to hold people accountable for their misfortune, to blame them, but I've learned that most of us are only a few bad breaks away from Mr. Green's three layers of pants. Over the years, he has revealed to me snippets of who he once was many lifetimes ago: the death of his young child, the end of a marriage, the loss of a job, the missed rent payments, the depression, and of course, the booze. Severe mental illness afflicts up to a quarter of all homeless people, so it's hard to gauge how much Mr. Green can help himself. Protecting him from the ravages of a bitter-cold night could save his life. Hypothermia is a preventable tragedy. It kills around 700 homeless or near homeless people in the United States each year. If I were in Mr. Green's shoes, I'd be curled up on an ER stretcher, too. The decision to hold Mr. Green until the morning isn't necessarily what good doctors do— it's what good neighbors do.

Sadly, emergency medicine trades in high volume misfortune, and there are many patients like Mr. Green in the ER. I'll grapple with such compassionate allocation decisions multiple times during the night. If there were plenty of ER beds, we could attend to patients with acute medical problems and make space for those with social ones. But there aren't.

Making clinical decisions under intense conditions where stress, urgency, interruptions, and uncertainty are the norm can produce giant cognitive headaches. The decisions are difficult, but they don't trap the heart in a hornet's nest, which is how this matter with Mr. Green feels. Making a compassionate decision for this patient means making a risky decision for the thirty patients in the waiting room.

My compassion must extend to them as well. They're not in rooms, but they're in our home. They have names and faces and concerns of their own.

Should Mr. Green be found frozen on the street after being discharged from the emergency department, or should a patient die because it took too long for her to be evaluated, there will be no shortage of critics. However, the pressures and conditions that led to these outcomes and the possibility that compassion, not insensitivity, might be partly to blame would likely receive less consideration.

Many of my colleagues would keep Mr. Green and the other homeless intoxicants until morning without a second thought. Their rationale: "I can't send Mr. Green or Mr. X or Ms. Y out into the street." When I remind them of the masses in the waiting room, they nod, a pained expression creases their face, and they shrug—what are we to do? Some are making a safer choice—allocating their compassion to the identifiable person under their care. For others, the possibility of bad things lurking in a sick waiting room patient is unfortunate, but discharging Mr. Green back into the cold in the middle of the night hits at a nerve that runs through the moral center of the medical profession.

We don't often talk about compassion as a justice problem. How do we allocate compassion to everyone who needs and deserves it fairly and equitably, especially when the choices lead to zero-sum gain—a win for one person must come as a loss for others? There's something called "compassion fatigue" in healthcare workers, which comes from constant contact with patients and their traumatic and stressful experiences. It's marked by symptoms that include apathy, depression, mistakes in clinical judgment, problems with sleep, and feelings of helplessness and anger. There's also compassion satisfaction, positive emotions that emerge from the act of caregiving. At moments such as this one with Mr. Green, my compassion doesn't grade onto this scale. It's neither exhausted nor a source of meaning. I suffer from compassion confusion.

I walk out to the waiting room's triage area and try to care for those patients who have relatively straightforward problems: swollen ankle, cough, medication refill. Problems that don't need prolonged workups and won't burden my nursing colleagues who are busy triaging the constant influx of new patients. As I walk among the swell of waiting people, some of whom might be quite sick, I'm frozen by their stares. I feel the urgency of their presence. The expectation in this sea of faces chills me as much as the harsh outside conditions. I want to care for these people as much as I want to care for Mr. Green.

I hear myself reasoning, doing the ugly work of balancing compassion with reality. Mr. Green already had access to our services. Discharging him into harsh conditions is risky, but I'm sending him back to his "normal" life, as abnormal and difficult as it might be. He must have nooks and crannies for keeping warm, right? Right? Typing these words now, years later, makes my skin crawl.

I've written about this situation previously, and I've received comments from readers calling me a cold, heartless physician. Indeed, there must be a place in the ER, in some hallway, to put these patients? I deserve their anger, fueled in part by their compassion for Mr. Green and others struggling to find a footing in a life that isn't fair.

When dealing with scarce resources, every effort should be made to increase capacity. If the pie isn't big enough for everyone, we must try to make a bigger pie. But when you're forced to work with a limited number of beds, other logistical factors like nurse–patient ratios, staffing, and safety concerns prevent us from letting Mr. Green camp out in the department while ushering in waiting patients.

Compassion reflects the culture of institutions. Compassionate operations acknowledge the suffering and distress of others—patients and staff—and make meaningful efforts to respond to them. Better yet, they shape strategies that prevent or minimize the possibility of people ever finding themselves in such untenable situations.

In this situation, my compassion stands speechless at the crossroads. To be moved by another's plight requires imagining and identifying with a sufferer. But I can only travel the emotional ground in one direction. Inevitably, there's a road not taken, one that can't be taken. Depending on where a bystander is situated, my actions may appear caring or cold.

I discharge Mr. Green. He's less upset than ornery and surprised that we woke him. He often goes back out to the waiting room, but tonight he's not interested. As I watch him take steady strides on his way out of the ER, I become unsteady and ashamed. Discussions around the lack of compassion in medicine must account for these gritty situations where more compassion isn't the solution.

An hour later, a different EMS crew rolls in with Mr. Green on a stretcher. Disheartened he's back, I'm also relieved he's safe. His alcohol level is four times than when he left, likely due to the alcohol he keeps stashed in places near the hospital. At least now, Mr. Green is out of the cold. And he'll wait. Waiting and warmth will stand for compassion, at least for the moment. Problems weren't solved but moved around, a perfect metaphor for how our health care system currently operates.

17

Pain: A Story That's Hard to Treat

Sonny D is cupping his jaw with both hands, writhing on the gurney, and pleading with me to give him "something for the pain." His teeth, those that remain, are a ragtag crew of decay. He's been popping ibuprofen like candy. Antibiotics no longer help. He needs a dentist, but he lacks insurance and the private dentists he contacted won't see him without cash up front. "I'm trying, doc," he says as if reading my mind. "You think I want to be here?"

I don't know what to think. Sonny wants what he says worked the last few times he came to the ER for dental pain. He's asking for Vicodin, a combination of the opioid hydrocodone and acetaminophen. Opioids—whether it's Vicodin or oxycodone or many others—have transformed the treatment of dental and other pain into a moral and clinical cage fight.

This struggle gets lost in the headlines. In 2014, there were 245 million prescriptions for opioids across the United States. An incredible and devastating amount, roughly one prescription for every adult. And data from the CDC show that four out of five heroin users began their habit by using prescription opioids, though these numbers have been contested. Looking at the statistics, it's easy to see why opioid deaths have quadrupled over the past three decades. But looking into Sonny's mouth makes my own jaw throb. In my ER practice, these statistics have faces, and sometimes these faces have rotted teeth, and these teeth can be a source of unbearable pain.

Will the opioid pills Sonny is asking for treat his pain, feed an addiction, or both? Will prescribing it fulfill a moral responsibility to alleviate his distress, contribute to the supply chain in the illicit pill economy, or both? Prescribing guidelines from the Centers for Disease Control and Prevention and recommendations from medical specialties and local hospitals are well intentioned and necessary. But they do little to address the central anxiety that makes this decision a source of distress for physicians like me. Treating Sonny D's pain is a narrative challenge as well as a medical one.

The physician/writer David Biro writes achingly about pain as a quintessentially private experience: "Pain of any variety isolates us from our family and closest friends. No one could feel what I felt during my transplant—not my wife or my parents or my sisters. And the inability to find words for my feelings only exacerbated my loneliness."

Pain is mysterious, different from almost everything else clinicians treat in medicine. Pain can't be dissected apart, located on a CT scan, or measured by a lab test. Its presence is undeniable to patients and hard to translate to others, posing a challenge to physicians and patients like Sonny D.

In her book *The Body in Pain*, Elaine Scarry says it best: "To have pain is to have certainty; to hear about pain is to have doubt." When the road into this private place is through the story the patient tells, my judgment of Sonny's pain will rely, in part, upon my judgment of his story.

Sonny tells me his pain is an 11, off the charts on the standard 1 to 10 pain scale. I have an image in my mind of distress that's beyond severe, and Sonny D isn't it. He's not screaming or moaning or writhing around. In 2001, the professed public health crisis in the United States was, allegedly, the undertreatment of pain. As part of its response, the Joint Commission wed farce with policy and declared pain a fifth vital sign. It didn't matter that pain possessed none of the measurable qualities shared by the other vital signs—pulse, blood pressure, breathing rate, and body temperature. Pain scales were instituted, and patients' self-reports were expected to be aggressively treated, often with opioids, a practice that fueled overprescribing and contributing to the opioid crisis. Assigning pain a number doesn't fully capture a complex experience, but because it's easier to comprehend, there's a tendency to regard the number as equivalent to the pain itself.

I have my doubts about Sonny. And I doubt my doubts. His medical record reveals multiple visits to the ER in the past few months, always in the heart of the night, for the same throbbing ache. Past treatment has included antibiotics, ibuprofen, naproxen, and opioids, though never for more than a few days.

He shakes off my suggestion of a local nerve block, the preferred remedy to numb dental pain. "They tried that the last time," he says. "The pain finds a way in."

Sonny needs a dentist, not opioids. I suggest phone numbers to local dental clinics.

"Called them," he says, "left messages. They don't call back. The clinics that answer the phone are booked for months."

I sympathize with Sonny. I sympathize with the overworked dental clinics. That said, every emergency physician has been duped by patients who use the ruse of pain to feed an addiction and divert drugs onto the streets. Decades of experience have created an internal radar for red-flag behaviors that raise the suspicion of "doctor shopping"—seeing multiple providers in hopes of finding one with a lower threshold for prescribing opioids. But I've discovered that this gut instinct is prone to error, again and again.

A good story engages our emotions and slips past our analytical neural circuitry, influencing our decisions and defying our better judgment. Research using fMRI shows how our brains respond to story—whether it's a movie or a story on the page—as if it's happening to us. In fact, a coupling develops between the speaker and listener, creating a synchronized neural activity that might be described as a shared brain. Researchers speculate that "dialogue will produce especially strong forms of synchronization." The stronger the connection between speaker and listener, the closer the coupling.

"Look at this mouth," says Sonny. "Is this the mouth of a faker? I used to be a good-looking guy."

I believe that. His T-shirt, an open flannel shirt, jeans, and steel-tipped work boots impart a rugged charm.

The tragic opioid data sits in the rational part of my brain. But population data must compete against one man's story of dental pain. And when a story gets its hooks in us, I get pulled into his story, become part of his experience. I have to ask myself, "What's my role here?" Am I a force for compassion or an agent of skepticism? A pain reliever or an addiction feeder? This is a complex question without a single answer. For example, compassion may push me to prescribe opioids, relieve his pain, and open up the possibility of addiction. What happens if I treat him with another method that hasn't been successful? The consequences of my actions are unknowable and unpredictable at this moment.

People who are swept away by a story begin to see the world in a manner consistent with the story. Once transported in this way, there's a tendency to let our guard down. Facts and data matter less than the quality and believability of the story. A well-told story with a dramatic arc can elicit empathy and influence our behavior by stimulating the release of the neurochemical oxytocin, which has ties to generosity, trustworthiness, and mother-infant bonding. I'm intrigued by the possibility that clinicians' vulnerability to deceit is often grounded in the empathy they are reported to be lacking.

I review the statewide prescription monitoring database. Sonny's name pops up and it aligns with his medical record: prescriptions for a few days of opioids here and there. But they are written by multiple healthcare providers, not one.

Such a pattern echoes the activity of someone hunting opioids for illicit purposes. I explain to Sonny that in an opioid epidemic, perception alone can harden into permanent suspicion. Even people without a prior history of abuse are at increased risk for developing opioid use disorder. The decision to expose Sonny's body to opioids requires balancing his present level of discomfort with the possibility of a future addiction.

"What about your medical doctor?" I ask Sonny. He shrugs. His medical clinic has a strict policy against prescribing opioids, another reason he's in the ER.

"I'm stuck," he says. "I know you probably don't believe me."

I'm stuck, too.

Sonny's story knocks against other stories I heard during that night's shift, such as the man complaining that he couldn't walk because of excruciating back pain who jumped off the stretcher and stormed out when we wouldn't prescribe Dilaudid, a powerful opioid painkiller.

I recognize that patients may get defensive when medical personnel doubt their stories. Implicit and explicit biases produce disturbing value judgments that result in inadequate and inexcusable responses to pain that contradict the medical profession's moral precept of "do no harm" and treat all patients with dignity and respect. For example, patients with sickle cell disease endure severe pain in their bones and describe experiences with medical staff that compound their suffering. Black and Hispanic ER patients are more likely than non-whites to receive no analgesia for extremity fractures. Studies show racial and ethnic disparities in opioid prescribing for conditions without objective findings, such as migraine and back pain. In the ER, where patients are "known" in snapshots of time, unfounded opinions and biases about patients don't always have a fair opportunity to be identified and corrected. Biases risk pushing further away patients who may already feel isolated in their pain.

Pain is modulated and given significance by the mind, but validated and afforded legitimacy by clinicians. When it comes to pain, which ear are clinicians listening with? The ear open to the investigation of pain, or the ear on the lookout for opioid-seeking behavior? Both ears must be recruited for this endeavor. However, patients might not trust clinicians when they have the impression they're speaking into a skeptic's ear.

My relationship to Sonny's pain deepens as I learn how he supports his young family by juggling two jobs. He works at a warehouse until 2 a.m. four nights a week. I ask Sonny how he could have been sleeping in the waiting room, his jean jacket pulled over his eyes, and then be rocking in pain in the examination area with 11 out of 10 pain. His wife came and waited with him in the emergency department for a few hours tonight. Before his wife left to get their kids off to school and head to work, he says she gave him some ibuprofen that took the edge off.

I'm curious how he endured the pain yesterday and the day before. And what about tomorrow? He lowers his head, assumes a posture of confession. Sometimes he buys Vicodin and other opioids on the street when the pain becomes unbearable. Besides being illegal, this business model is rife with quality control problems. I've lost count of the number of accidental overdoses where patients thought they were buying one drug and we later find out, or the coroner does, that it was cut with fentanyl, a potent synthetic opioid that can be up to a hundred times more powerful than morphine.

Sure, alternatives to opioids are ideal. Examples include regional nerve blocks, disease-specific therapies, and an integrative approach to pain. They aren't risk-free, but medical decision-making is always a wrestling match between risks and benefits. With Sonny, however, I can't dodge the opioid question.

Overdoses and substance abuse are a devastating part of my practice. But without a dental appointment in sight, Sonny will be back, incurring the financial burden of another ER visit. Or he'll find what he needs on the street. If Sonny comes to the ER in pain and goes home in pain, what does that say about me? I've perpetrated a grave moral harm. Not only because I provided substandard care, but because at the heart of all, I didn't believe him and I didn't completely trust what he was saying.

Stories serve as instruments for connection as well as tools of deception. The paradox of responsible pain management involves finding compassionate ways to curb opioid prescribing while not curbing the clinician's interest in the patient's experience of pain. And if opioids are a problem, we need to think about addiction as a narrative to be understood rather than a habit to be judged.

Story can empower patients by making them heroes in their own stories. Clinicians must learn to offer every patient an affirmation of their struggles, and recognize how difficult life can be in the throes of pain. In his book *The Culture of Pain*, David Morris states that to be in pain is to be in a state of crisis: modern medicine, with its Western, technocratic worldview, misrepresents pain as purely a medical problem, the creation of anatomy and physiology, and ignores the experience of pain as phenomena of the mind, shaped by historical, cultural, and psychosocial factors.

In an opioid crisis, it can be hard for clinicians to think of the experience of pain as a crisis, too. It's easier to simplify the experience than amplify it, build an inventory that categorizes the pain—throbbing, burning, or aching—and quantifies it with a number on a pain scale, then dive into its impact and meaning in a patient's life. Pain can influence relationships, job performance, and the ability to think and reflect clearly. Pain integrates into a person's identity, affecting their ability to function in the present and their capacity to envision a better future.

The people impacted by the tragedy of the opioid crisis have stories to tell, too. So do those patients suffering from pain. We need all their stories, including those from clinicians struggling to navigate these choppy waters responsibly. And what can't be ignored is the tragic story of dental care inequality. In the United States, many people suffer from mouth disease, endure pain, and risk medical complications due to lack of insurance or inadequate coverage. Just as I find pain scales absurd for their false objectivity, I find pretending that definitive help is on the way for Sonny D a false possibility.

Relieving pain is a basic human gesture, and yet in an opioid crisis a simple case of dental pain becomes a major dilemma. I prescribe a few doses of Vicodin for Sonny. I can't say I made the right decision. But indifference isn't a virtue, and writing prescriptions for medications that haven't been effective doesn't feel right either. I wasn't just responding to his pain, but to his struggles, of which the pain is a part. Responsible pain management can't rely on pain scales alone. We must be willing to dignify the storyteller and travel with them into their story.

18
There's Dying, and Dying Now

The two medics pushing Mrs. M into the ER are sweating more than she is, and she's gulping after every oxygen molecule inside the oxygen mask. Her chest heaves and caves. "Hi, Mrs. M." She opens her eyes. But her glassy stare lands beyond me. "She has metastatic lung cancer," says one of the medics. My heart suddenly feels heavy. "She's in hospice," says the medic. My relief is audible. The medic then shakes his head. "But her son wants everything done."

"Doing everything isn't a plan compatible with hospice," I say.

"She wasn't this bad when we arrived at her home," says the medic. "She was working pretty hard, but not like this."

Hospice care provides a team-oriented approach to patients with a terminal disease who have less than six months to live. The goal is compassionate end-of-life care. The focus is controlling pain and other distressing symptoms and meeting the emotional and spiritual needs of patients and their family members. Hospice services allow patients to live out their final days at home and die with dignity, not in hospitals receiving invasive and often painful tests and procedures that often prolong the dying process.

That should have been what happened with Mrs. M. But her son called 911 and now she is in the ER. I ask the medics for any hospice-related paperwork. They raise empty hands. There's no advance directive or MOLST (medical orders for life-sustaining treatment) form, either, meaning no documentation telling me what kind of end-of-life care Mrs. M wanted—or didn't want.

"Is her son here?" I ask.

They point to the hallway outside the exam room.

Paul is a thin, nervous man with a windbreaker still zipped to his throat. In a trembling voice, he describes how his mother felt weak and tired throughout the day. Then the evening came, and her breathing got suddenly worse.

"Please doctor, do something," he says.

It's neither a request nor a demand. It's a plea that contains a quiet emotional force and presumes we share a common understanding on one key point: what that "something" is.

I must take some definitive action very soon. Usually, the lungs take in oxygen and expel carbon dioxide. Monitors show that not enough oxygen is reaching Mrs. M's bloodstream, and carbon dioxide is building up, rising to dangerous levels. A portable chest X-ray reveals lungs overrun with cancer and a bank of clouds suggesting pneumonia.

Although most Americans say they want to die at home, many die in hospitals. Multiple factors account for this, including challenges related to end-of-life planning and communication. A practical and meaningful process requires several elements to be in place. Patients must discuss their goals of care with family members and healthcare providers.

These wishes and discussions must be documented, kept up to date, and made available to emergency providers like me who, confronted with hard decisions under pressing time constraints, are desperate for guidance.

When a patient ceases to have the capacity to make decisions, a designated surrogate, which I assume is Paul, is entrusted with making decisions as the patient would have, meaning consistent with their wishes and goals. But over the years, I've observed how even the most loving, informed, and prepared surrogates may appear knocked off balance when that moment finally comes.

I explain to Paul that his mother will die if I don't insert a breathing tube into her airway and connect her to a ventilator. He nods. He's aware that his mother is terminally ill with metastatic cancer, that it's irreversible, and intervening with a breathing tube won't change that. He confirms her wishes, agrees that she wanted hospice care. Then says: "Do everything."

I bite my lip and quickly turn away.

I ask if he understands what hospice means. Back in medical school, a VA patient with end-stage lung cancer taught me an invaluable lesson about assuming a patient understands the terms doctors use. He was actively dying, and despite multiple discussions with various senior physicians on the treatment team, he refused to sign an advance directive. His presumed stubbornness frustrated the team, who believed resuscitation would be futile. I asked an intern who wasn't directly involved with his care for advice. This was his suggestion: ask him what he thinks DNR ("do not resuscitate") means. Before the patient kicked me out of his room, I posed that very question. He stopped his yelling. Tears watered his eyes. "It means you'll stop caring for me." He didn't want a breathing machine or CPR or any aggressive treatments. He wasn't scared of death; he was terrified of dying. "Doing everything" was his hedge against perceived abandonment.

Paul nods. "Please do everything, doctor," he says.

Heat beams from my eyeballs. But he seems so fragile. I worry that my frustration will only upset him. But I have a dying, barely responsive patient who cannot speak for herself and a family member begging for treatment that contradicts her wishes to the best of my knowledge. Medications aren't working. And she's too sleepy for a BIPAP mask, a form of noninvasive ventilation for acute respiratory failure that might otherwise buy us time.

Mrs. M weighs more than three hundred pounds. She has a short neck of multiple chins, and when I quickly check under the oxygen mask, I find a small mouth. These physical attributes are important because it will likely be a challenge to pass a breathing tube down her throat. The nurse I am working with shoots me a look—that look, a wordless kick in the ass. We don't have time.

I describe what "doing everything" involves. We will first try to intubate her, which means putting a breathing tube down her throat and into her airway, then connect it to a machine that will breathe for her. If we can't intubate her, we will need to cut into her neck with a scalpel and insert the breathing tube below her vocal cords, called a cricothyroidotomy. If her heart stops, we'll press on her chest. Sometimes, the compressions break ribs.

Paul scrunches his face as if defending himself from my explanation. I don't want to be gruesome, but I've witnessed the gulf between words and actions. I remember one particular situation when a patient's daughter wouldn't let me end resuscitation efforts after her father cycled in and out of cardiac arrest for over an hour. His prognosis was dismal. The family assembled in a family room just off the treatment area. Finally, I asked if she'd like to see what we were doing. As soon as she stepped into the resuscitation room she dropped to her knees and screamed "Stop! What are you doing?"

The same interventions that are life-saving and critical in certain situations can be viewed as cruel and unnecessary treatment for someone who likely wants comfort measures only. It also puts the physicians and nurses caring for Mrs. M in a morally distressing position.

I detail the comfort care we would provide Paul's mother if we honor her wishes. It includes giving her oxygen, controlling her pain, and using medications to mitigate her dyspnea, or air hunger. The goals of those kinds of care—to relieve suffering—are different, but we would be just as aggressive as if we were "doing everything."

The care will continue.

"We're staying right here," I tell Paul. "We won't leave your mother alone."

He suggests we wait. He needs to talk to his sister. It's almost 2 a.m., and she's at work.

I shake my head. Indecision is the worst possible decision. "She's coming," says Paul. "She should be here in an hour."

An emergency physician is trained to save lives. But when a patient at the end of their life wishes for a comfortable death, that becomes my goal, too. That opportunity usually comes along only once, and this chance is slipping away. Advance directives speak for us when we lose the mental capacity to speak for ourselves. They chronicle our values and beliefs, what brings us joy, the burdens we're willing to endure for an acceptable quality of life, and when we would want to refuse or stop treatment.

The Patient Self-Determination Act, implemented in 1991, requires healthcare institutions to give you a written summary of your healthcare decision-making rights, ask if you have an advance directive, and document the answer in your medical record. Sadly, the cherished idea of respecting patient autonomy and preserving dignity at the end of life by providing cogent directions to health care providers like me hasn't translated well into practice.

MOLST or POLST (physician orders for life-sustaining treatment) programs hold promise as medical orders that communicate specific preferences for patients facing life-limiting illnesses. However, these documents may contain confusing or even contradictory instructions that physicians must interpret at a time of crisis when clarity is needed. For example, a form indicates a patient doesn't want any resuscitative efforts and desires a "natural death only" but also expresses no limits on medical interventions, which implies "do everything."

What may seem to be contradictory instructions could reflect challenges inherent in predicting unforeseen situations. A patient with congestive heart failure may ask not to have CPR if her heart suddenly stops, but may want a time-limited trial of intubation if her lungs fill with fluid because that condition might be reversible.

A healthcare surrogate, usually a family member, is supposed to make the same decisions the patient would have made if they could do so. But surrogates incorrectly predict patient preferences approximately one-third of the time. I ask surrogates to pretend their loved one suddenly became lucid and understood their present situation—what would they want?

I'm not sure what Paul understands. Sometimes family members are overwhelmed by making potentially life-changing decisions for their critically ill loved ones. The experience can produce profound emotional consequences later on. I've cared for families who choose doing everything possible not only out of fear of being abandoned, but for reasons unrelated to the medical issues. For example, siblings and relatives will blame them for "killing" mom and they'll shoulder this burden for the rest of their lives.

Though I'm horrified by the possibility of performing life-saving measures on a patient who has expressed other preferences, I'm not in a position to unilaterally decide "doing everything" is inappropriate.

I'm unable to contact Paul's sister. I can't convince myself that Mrs. M isn't deteriorating quickly. We can't find hospice paperwork. I intubate her.

The breathing tube slips in easily. I want to collapse with joy. For the moment, Mrs. M is stable and sedated. The ventilator is breathing for her, preventing her from dying from respiratory failure. But now I'm distressed. Intubating her feels wrong, though necessary given the circumstances.

Finally, I have a chance to dive into Mrs. M's medical records. The electronic medical record should make advance care planning information more accessible. In emergency settings, urgency might not allow us to dig through a patient's chart. I'm dumbfounded that this information is often not readily available, even among older patients with significant medical problems.

I'm grateful to find a note in the record from Mrs. M's oncologist. Earlier in the week this doctor discussed Mrs. M's prognosis with her. She likely had months to live. Mrs. M refused any further chemotherapy and said she didn't want to be intubated or receive CPR. It was at this visit that her oncologist referred her to hospice care. The note also alluded to difficult conversations with the family, who were less accepting of Mrs. M's prognosis than she was.

The wording implied the family presented an obstacle. I'm not absolved of such judgments. I was clearly frustrated with Paul. But if this indeed was true, why would they think this way? It might be read as an unwillingness to accept the prognosis. But to accept something, one must consent to receive it. What if their "problem" was a problem in how the information was delivered? The family's perceived inability to accept her prognosis may have had more to do with their distrust of the healthcare system or with physicians in general.

Paul's sister, Violet, finally arrives. She's dressed in scrubs, having rushed over from her job as a certified nursing assistant in a nursing home. There's an intensity in the way she slings her handbag over her shoulder and listens as I share with her and Paul what I read in her mother's medical record, including direct comments from the oncologist. I'm glad she's in the medical field. I assume I have an ally in this dilemma, that we share a common understanding about the moral force of advance directives. Violet nods attentively, then insists that we keep her mother on the ventilator.

"Please?" she asks.

The ventilator breathing for Mrs. M feeds oxygen while blowing off the excess carbon dioxide, which accumulated as a result of her respiratory failure and was primarily responsible for her somnolence. As the carbon dioxide level in her bloodstream drops, she slowly emerges into wakefulness. I was going to increase her sedation, but her eyes open to Violet's voice and she gestures to pull out the breathing tube.

"She wants to talk," Violet says.

"To do that, I'll have to take out the tube," I say.

"We know she's dying," Violet says, her teary eyes turning to her mom. "We were hoping for a little more time."

I have heard this many times from families. Their expectations might seem unrealistic, but they're doing their best to keep death in the future. There is a profound difference between the idea of dying when death is an omnipresent shadow on some distant horizon and when it is happening right now.

We give Mrs. M morphine to make her comfortable and remove the breathing tube. She's alert enough to share kisses with Violet and Paul. We pull chairs into the room, and her family gathers around her stretcher.

"She raised us all by herself," says Violet, holding her mother's hand. "She worked every day, I mean every day, to support us. She's the toughest woman you'll ever meet."

I look at Paul, sitting beside his mother and rubbing her arm. Of course, he was going to insist on doing everything— what the oncologist and providers like me consider compassionate care is, in his mind, giving up.

Sister and brother collapse into each other's arms. I take over holding Mrs. M's hand, part comfort, part apology for what I'd done. I could have framed the discussion differently, recognizing their mother's wishes and supporting their emotional needs as decision-makers.

In a 1995 article, bioethicist Daniel Callahan wrote, "Is death a friend or an enemy, to be acquiesced to or to be fought?" He said that the US healthcare system isn't sure how to answer that question. I think the same holds for most families.

A peace descends on the room. Paul and Violet sit holding her hand, fixing a stray hair. Her nurse lowers the lights and shuts off the monitor. I take a deep breath, grateful that Mrs. M received a second chance at a good death.

19
Holding On, Letting Go

I cried when Pivo, our fourteen-year-old Cocker-King Cavalier mix, raised a trembling leg to piss on the Bradford pear and tumbled over. He sniffed around a little more on this cool, spring morning. Then we drove him to the vet and put him to sleep.

As an ER doctor with experience in medical ethics, I thought I was prepared for his end-of-life struggles. But that knowledge didn't prevent me from hitting the same familiar obstacles I've pointed out to families of dying ER patients for decades. Understanding Pivo's suffering at the end of his life was difficult not because we couldn't ask him—though that's part of it—but because our hope kept getting in the way.

An instrument hasn't been invented to measure hope, assure us our hope is appropriate and appropriately dosed, and warn us when it turns selfish. With Pivo, our worry ran on a spectrum. Were we giving up too soon or holding on too long? Despite our iron commitment to minimizing his suffering, the solidity of our judgments was less reliable.

I'm not implying our pets are equivalent to our spouses, partners, children, and others we love. But pets often feel like family members. "It's a dog's life" is a common expression. But what is a dog's life? And how would we know an unacceptable dog's life? How much easier it would be if he could tell us, "I'm ready."

We thought the fateful moment arrived a year earlier. Pivo's arthritis made standing on all fours a losing fight with gravity. Before long, we were carrying him up and down the stairs. At first, he growled at being lifted. The indignity of such assistance, we thought—or it could be the pain we were causing his lumpy and sore-riddled body in the name of help. Eventually, he settled into our arms, and we wondered if his surrender was a signal that we misinterpreted as gratitude.

We tailored each ominous moment into an optimistic story. A new dog food for his weight loss. A new medication would provide more energy, or maybe his sluggishness was a side effect of the drug for his pain. He'd slide down a few steps before catching himself on the hardwood stairs he once sprung up and down with abandon, yet we'd focus on a recent instance when he handled the stairs slowly, but without incident. His tailed wagged when he played with the other dogs. He must be experiencing pleasure or excitement if his tail still wags.

Suffering is a personal experience that's difficult to penetrate. The perception and purpose of suffering differ across cultures, religions, and groups around the globe—not to mention the leap between species. Victor Frankl, the famed psychiatrist and Holocaust survivor, described suffering as an opportunity for achievement. Frankl wrote, "If there is a meaning in life at all, then there must be a meaning in suffering." But this empowering dimension to suffering may have unintended consequences, giving people who don't share this viewpoint another cause to suffer. In the documentary *How to Die in Oregon*, a film about the Death with Dignity Act, which granted terminally ill people the right to self-administer medications to end their life, a dying patient asks: "Do you think it's cowardice not to want to suffer?"

We visited the vet several times for her wisdom. We didn't want him to suffer, but we weren't ready to let him go. He spent more days sprawled on his belly, his legs twitching. The ledger of suffering and debilitation were adding up week by week, and yet we always found reasons for hope. Until one day, when he hurled down the entire stairs, bouncing and sliding on his back until he struck the landing. He popped up quickly, too quickly, almost as if making a statement about his toughness. But he was panting, shaking, flashing a look that we interpreted as terror.

There was no way to know what was racing through his mind, but we couldn't escape the thoughts flying through ours. He would die soon, regardless of whether we were ready to let him go. What if he were severely injured from the fall down the staircase? What if we weren't home, and he endured hours of pain from a broken bone or internal injury? What if he died scared and alone?

Minimizing suffering is a critical factor in this decision, but so is the preservation of dignity. In studies that looked into why patients in Oregon decided to end their life, the most common were loss of autonomy, no longer finding enjoyment in pleasurable activities, loss of dignity, and pain. Maybe we went too far imparting human feelings onto a dog, but Pivo was a lumpy, smelly member of our family. We discovered a merciful death was an idea easy to embrace and easier to get wrong. The grief of letting go bumped against the worry of giving up too soon and the fear we had waited too long.

His eyes shut after the vet pushed the barbiturate through the intravenous in his leg. We held tight, felt his weight soften as we lowered him to his dog bed, where we often found him, his head perched, his tail wagging.

20
When Waiting Feels Immoral

Mr. Kane uses one hand to clutch the plastic basin into which he is vomiting and gesturing hello with the other hand when I introduce myself in the ER triage area.

He has suffered from headaches ever since he had surgery for a brain mass years before. The pain, described as a hot knife behind his eyes, is typically controlled with over-the-counter medication. But he's vomiting the pain pills. I examine him, start treatment, and tag him for an urgent bed in the main ER.

Only there aren't any beds immediately available. So, he'll be sent back into the waiting room in the company of the many other waiting patients, some possibly sicker than he is.

"This is wrong!" Mrs. Kane lashes out. Her tone cuts me and the nursing staff. She wants nothing to do with my apologies. Words won't make her husband better.

Mrs. Kane takes her cell phone and starts calling for an ambulance to take him to another hospital. She attracts the attention of other aggrieved patients in the triage room—people unnerved that they've been waiting, too. They're now curious onlookers. Desperate to appease the Kanes and explain what we can do to make him more comfortable until a bed opens up, I fear these other patients might behave similarly.

Emergency medicine is firmly grounded in social justice and providing access to expert care to everyone who comes in. Treating anyone, with any condition, at any time is ideal. But most ERs don't enjoy a limitless supply of beds and staff to treat everyone at the same time. Patient prioritization uses a system that might be perceived as unjust: the concept of triage. The emergency queue isn't necessarily "first come, first served." It's nonlinear by design, with a focus on illness severity. The severely ill or injured receive immediate attention and everyone else, to various degrees, must wait. Though studies cast an ugly shadow on notions of "objective" triage assessments by highlighting the influence of racial and gender bias.

When too many ER beds are occupied with boarded patients (i.e., patients waiting for an inpatient hospital bed to become available), flow backs up to the triage area, where patients will tell you exactly how they feel about the perceived injustice. The pressure in this narrow clinical area builds. It's more than their frustration. It's the strain of shouldering the blame and the burden of their outrage, especially when I have little, if any, control over larger system issues. It's situations like this one when waiting feels immoral.

Waiting is the action of remaining where one is or delaying action until a future time when something else happens. Waiting in the ER isn't only a stressful test of endurance. It's a first-order oxymoron. Just as the word "waiting" seems out of place in a sentence that includes "emergency," the concept of a waiting room feels wrong in a space dedicated to treating emergencies. But a bustling ER waiting room is a warped and inescapable reality in hospitals.

Because of Mr. Kane's history of a brain mass, severe pain, and constant wrenching, the nurses bump him ahead in the queue, which upsets some patients who have been waiting much longer. When I try to point this out to Mrs. Kane, I detect a blend of appreciation and dissatisfaction. It isn't enough. Her expectations, I understand, are both reasonable and unreasonable, given the circumstances. "Look at him," she says.

I nod, recognizing his misery. But I also want to nod toward the other patients and acknowledge their needs, too. Those skipped over are rarely happy about it. The perception of fairness shapes people's impression of waiting. I want to say to Mrs. Kane that we're trying our best, only I've learned to use these words cautiously when people clearly disapprove of your "best." It also suggests that perhaps we're unwilling or unable or lack the necessary imagination to do more.

"What are you doing for my husband?" Mrs. Kane asks. I ordered medications for his pain and vomiting to be given by mouth since patients can't go back into the waiting room with IVs. But chances are he vomited these meds. He wipes his mouth with a towel as I reexamine him. Bloodwork sent; he needs IV fluids and intravenous medications. He deserves better than this modified version of our best.

Each time Mr. Kane vomits serves as a reminder that I'm an agent at the gate of waiting.

My aggravation needs an exhaust valve, so I become short-tempered with hard-working staff who are doing their best, too. I swing into the triage rooms of other patients and apologize for the wait. One woman screams at me and the interpreter in Spanish, and she has every right to scream. She came to the ER the night before but left because she couldn't wait any longer. Wherever I move in the triage area, Mrs. Kane appears, increasingly upset. Excuse me, doctor? How are we doing, doctor? Soon, I'm unable to contain my exasperation any longer.

"Please!" I say to her. "We know your husband is sick. We're working on beds. We're not going to let him stay this uncomfortable."

She throws me a suspicious look.

"I won't talk you out of your rage," I say. "You deserve it. It might not look like it, but we're on your side."

It's hard to bear the anger and frustration of patients and their families because you know you'd be complaining if you were in their situation. If the department's techs and nurses could fold an origami bed out of paper, they would gladly do that for Mr. Kane and the others.

ER crowding is a national problem described as a sign of an unhealthy hospital system that is associated with worse health outcomes. The ongoing pandemic amplified the crowding problem for many of us, often to excessive degrees, owing to illness severity, longer inpatient stays for COVID-19 patients, and staffing shortages. Before the pandemic, many hospitals instituted changes to cut wait times for emergency care, including moving doctors into the triage process to reduce the time to an evaluation by a physician. Our department has implemented this new vertical model, but its success depends on the freedom of downstream hospital bottlenecks.

Unfortunately, even on the best of days, a measure of waiting is part of the ER experience, even when we believe the patient is no longer waiting. After the patient is seen by a provider there's the wait for tests to be done followed by the wait for results. There's a wait for consultants to return our calls. We wait for social workers and case managers because patients bring a web of social issues, too. The wait for admission leads to waiting for a bed to become available and housekeeping to clean those beds. We focus on time whenever we think about the problem of waiting, but the experience of waiting is more complicated than a ticking clock.

Waiting is a potent form of inactivity. It can push us to exhaustion—"I'm tired of waiting"—and compel us to impetuous behavior. Who hasn't darted into the shorter supermarket line or nosed into the emptier lane on the highway only to be slowed down again? Waiting can distort the experience of time. Researchers in waiting, or queuing, say that our perception of waiting can feel as much as one-third longer than it is. In the ER, the perception of the wait contributes to patient dissatisfaction more than the actual wait.

Pioneers in wait management, the folks who run the Disney parks understand how to navigate expectations. Through distraction and constant entertainment, kids and parents are less aware of time's passing. So, a thirty-minute delay feels like a win when you expect forty-five.

But distraction is difficult when your fears will still be there after the distraction is over. The wait for a thrilling amusement park ride is not the same as waiting while tired, scared, hurt, and sick enough to warrant a detour from your daily routine for a trip to the ER. Frontline providers take a patient's presence in the ER for granted. But the decision to visit or call 911 isn't one that's taken lightly by most people. Their emotional states are as important as their chief complaint. As a result, many patients are strung tight when they arrive. Should they find further resistance in a long wait, or are plucked the wrong way by the wrong words or attitude from staff, they're primed to snap.

We must recognize that behind the waiting time is a blank stare, and behind that is a churning imagination.

The tense atmosphere in ER waiting rooms can feel like being lost in the Bermuda Triangle of might, should, and could. Patients bring with them more than symptoms and problems. Added to concerns about what might be causing their troubles are unmet desires and ideas about what should be happening—receiving medical attention. Life continues outside the hospital, spiking the wait with all that patients could be doing: earning money for rent and food, caring for an ill parent, picking up kids from school, feeding the dog, even sleeping. Strategies to reduce waiting times must not ignore the fact that patients might be adrift in some stressful and frightening places while they appear to be calmly sitting in a stiff chair.

Waiting is a universal experience and it ignites frustration in most, if not all, of us. In the ER, I've learned that waiting can serve as an occasion that unites patients, families, emergency physicians, and staff. Mrs. Kane was apoplectic, but despite her well-earned fury she could see our attempts to work within the existing constraints. I believe what finally calmed her was nothing we said, but recognizing through our actions that we were allies, that her fight was our fight.

There were no immediate beds in the ER proper for Mr. Kane. The techs and nurses found a space for him on a gurney in a part of the triage area. There are no columns on spreadsheets that capture the value of these silent gestures. Mrs. Kane was satisfied that we were keeping him in our sights. Mr. Kane could wait and be cared for. Which makes you wonder if it still counts as waiting. The data will show a long wait before he made it to a room, but the truth is that caring began soon after his arrival.

Mrs. Kane disrupted the triage area, but she also shook us up in a constructive way. Many of our patients didn't have family members advocating for them. We make a point to check in with everyone else we'd seen in the triage area and sent back to the waiting room so they, too, understand they are in our sights.

As the medications take effect, Mr. Kane stops vomiting and sinks into sleep. A quiet settles over the baseline turbulence in the triage area. Mrs. Kane holds the vomit basin that tilts precariously beside her husband's chest on the gurney. It seems too heavy for her arms. "We're glad he's feeling better," I say, sharing the news that thanks to the magic of nurses, a bed is targeted for him as soon as it's cleaned. She suddenly appears lost, exhausted. I fear she'll collapse, and soon we'll be treating her, too.

She opens up about all they'd gone through. Mr. Kane's surgeries, the onerous physical therapy, their kids in middle school, the long stretches when her husband was unable to work and the months when she couldn't work because she needed to care for him. Whenever he gets like this, she can't help but panic and fear the worst: the tumor is back.

Fear was the animating force behind Mrs. Kane's anger. The intensity of anger can force others on the receiving end to defend and react instead of interrogating the source of the anger, which is often fear. Anger is described as the "fight" part of the fight-or-flight response. Anger is such psychologically complex behavior. As she stood beside his stretcher watching him sleep, I saw a terrified wife and mother who would do anything for her husband and her family.

I've heard comments from patients and family surprised that we become as upset about their waiting as they were. How often have I fought the chasm between the care I should be providing and the watered-down version we could muster and craved for someone to yell at with Mrs. Kane's relentless fire.

In recent years, authors have coined the term "moral injury" to describe the agonizing compromises healthcare providers must make in their practice to satisfy an unhealthy and broken health system. These "betrayals of patient care and trust" take their toll. I leave hectic ER shifts that function well feeling beat up but invigorated. I leave shifts such as this one desperate to leave the practice of medicine.

We can measure time with a degree of accuracy, but responses to waiting are unique and unpredictable. I remember trying to reason with a patient with chronic knee pain who watched the ER staff rush into a room where a patient was in cardiac arrest. She saw us talking with the tearful family, the priest providing comfort outside the doorway. And yet she gave me an earful about how long she had to wait. The widening fissures in our social fabric and the glaring health inequities mean even the perception of injustice can justifiably provoke feelings of abandonment and push people to behaviors that shock their calmer selves. Most of the time, I'm astounded by the understanding offered by waiting patients and their family. Occasionally, I find patients come prepared with thick books in their hands. I hope you didn't expect to read five hundred pages, I say, taking in the doorstop of a novel in their laps.

Early in my emergency medicine training, a senior physician offered this bit of advice: When you enter a patient's room for the first time, introduce yourself and apologize for the wait, even if they've waited only five minutes. I rolled my eyes. It felt scripted, a patient satisfaction gimmick. But an apology recognizes that coming to the ER is hard and rife with emotion and that at that moment any wait is too long.

21
Benefit Paradox

"My ex calls 911 with some bull that I'm suicidal," said Mr. Atkins. "Next thing I know the police are pulling me out of bed."

"It's a tough world," I said. "I can't disagree with you."

I spoke too quickly. Insensitive and I knew it.

A worried nurse pulled me away to speak with Mr. Atkins, who was tired of waiting and wanted to leave. She was uncomfortable with that idea. The police were called for reports of depression and suicidal ideation.

"But I was sleeping," he said. "I work at 8 a.m. I'll be fired if I'm not there."

"I'm sorry." I held out my hand, introduced myself. He kept his hands buried in the pockets of his hoodie.

"Is that it?" he said.

"What did you expect?" I said.

"Another line of bull." His face, shaven and sunburnt, was set in a frozen stare.

"Not from me," I said. "Not tonight."

I'd been dealing with two sick patients and a guy known for his substance use who wouldn't leave the ER unless I wrote a narcotic script for his chronic back pain. Whatever empathy that remained in my pockets amounted to loose change. I invested all of it into Mr. Atkins, but the words still sounded second-hand and a bit tired. Even so, he said he appreciated my directness.

"Do you feel you might hurt yourself?" I asked.

I noticed his hands, stuffed into the front hand-warmers of the hoodie, fidgeting about.

"I never said that," he said. "For no good reason my ex tells me I can't see my kid this weekend. Three weeks of these games. I told her if I can't see him, I might as well be dead."

"Those words trigger responses," I said.

"But that was earlier. Why call 911 in the middle of the night? She's nuts. Please let me go."

He worked construction and the money he earned was already spent—child support for his ten-year-old son. He was prescribed antidepressants but couldn't afford them because he doesn't have health insurance. He met with a psychiatric social worker until her office hours jarred with the steady construction work the past six months. He was male, single, divorced, lonely, financially strapped. He wore red flags of suicide risk like a crown of thorns.

He was also future oriented, an adoring father hell-bent on regaining his financial footing.

"Please, doc. My sucky situation will suck more if my ass isn't on site at 08:00."

The decision to let him leave rested on certain critical questions: Is Mr. Atkins an imminent danger to himself? Is his untreated mental illness unstable at this moment? And what to make of his family stresses? He'd made an impulsive statement. Mr. Atkins didn't deny it. But are they empty words spoken too quickly, or are they signals that foreshadow an impulsive action in the immediate future?

It's not uncommon for people to be brought to the ER after making statements like "I want to kill myself" or "I'd rather be dead." Frequently, they're said in the heat of the moment, the heat fueled by alcohol or cocaine or other substances and often in response to a deep hurt, a violation of trust, a loss of control. Certain situations immediately come to mind: a break-up with a partner, a discovery of infidelity, a loss of a job and steady income, an overwhelmed and underappreciated caregiver. Frequently, patients under the influence of alcohol or drugs retract these statements when the substances leave their bloodstream and they've had a chance to sleep and calm down. However, our level of concern heightens when other features are in the picture, such as a history of serious mental illness, previous psychiatric hospitalizations, prior suicide attempts, and guns in the home.

Suicide sadly ranks as a leading cause of death. But many people who commit suicide don't want to die. They want to end their pain. They feel hopeless and helpless and even worthless. Suicide is often impulsive and a response to a momentary crisis. Was Mr. Atkins experiencing such a crisis?

Aspects of his story speak to his responsibility—a job, a kid he loves. If I found myself in his turbulent situation, I'd probably be upset, too. Then again, an understandable response in certain situations can turn extreme in others.

My head told me to let him walk. My gut said not so fast. I'm on justified ground holding him against his wishes for a more formal and expert evaluation by a psychiatric specialist if he poses a risk to self or others. But the psychiatric evaluation might not happen until morning. Mr. Atkins will miss work, join the unemployed, and sink deeper into financial troubles. By "helping" him, I might contribute to his future risk for suicide. And yet, he's also at risk if his earlier statements carried more weight than he was letting on. Each possibility forged shadowy figures in my mind, each distant but distinct enough to warrant my attention.

I felt yoked in a benefit paradox. The right thing to do wasn't clear. Both decisions may result in Mr. Atkins taking his life. From a medical-legal perspective, the easier decision is to hold him. His desire to hurt himself is documented in the record. But was what I might call prudence a disguise for lack of moral courage? What was at the core of my reluctance to let him leave: an unwillingness to absorb a small measure of uncertainty and a degree of risk, or were my doubts founded in deeper justifiable concerns about him?

"Mr. Atkins," I said. "Do you feel safe?"

"I live in a shelter. Not the safest place. That's why my ex doesn't want me to see my son."

I bit my lip.

"And my child support pays her rent."

My impression of him was constantly shifting. He wasn't a difficult patient. He was a difficult story. I asked if I might call his ex-wife to better flesh out what concerned her enough to call the police. It's not that I don't believe him, but it is one side of the story. He recoiled as if I'd just yanked off a scab. He refusal was so raw, I didn't push it further. He just wanted to get to work, that's all, and retreated into his hoodie.

"Please, doc," he said, looking over my shoulder to the wall clock.

Despite everything he was saying, there were words I wasn't hearing. He never stated explicitly that he no longer wanted to hurt himself.

I explained the value of keeping him for an evaluation by the psychiatrist, that we don't always realize we're inside a depression until we're out of it and looking back. The psychiatrist could help arrange counseling that might work better with his job and restart psychiatric medications.

"If I have a job."

"I'll write you a work note," I told him.

"Thanks, doc. My foreman will wipe his ass with it."

"Any family or friends who might float you some cash?"

"My father was born with a gold spoon."

"Have you asked him?"

Sometimes I hear myself asking questions so stupid and obvious, I break into a sweat.

"He's generous when it comes to throwing my failures in my face, but cheap with money."

I detected a shift in his posture, an ever-so-slight roll of the shoulders, an agitated rustling of his hands in the pockets.

"I get the sense that I should be worrying about you," I said.

"A man works for twenty-five years shouldn't be living in a shelter. I should have my own roof."

"Mr. Atkins?"

"But I'm not ashamed. Anything for my kid."

"Mr. Atkins," I said, leaning in so our eyes are level. "Do you have a plan?"

"I don't have health insurance if that's what you're asking."

I sat stone-faced. I must confess a certain admiration for his intelligent evasions even as they tested my patience. He was charming, the kind of person you find yourself rooting for. But I wasn't smiling. He ran his calloused fingers through his hair, neatly trimmed and peppered with gray. The silence was uncomfortable.

"I'd jump off a bridge," he said. The edge to his voice then softened. "If only I wasn't afraid of heights."

What a beautifully tilted line, especially from someone withholding his suicidal intentions.

"Have you ever tried to hurt yourself?"

He wouldn't answer.

"It's important to know."

"Never."

"Have you thought about it?"

He pushed his left hand beyond the ribbed sleeve cuffs. His answer a few beats behind my question, enough of a delay to imply that he wasn't responding but casually offering information. "Until last week," he said. Superficial cuts lined his wrist, as well as a deeper wound that would have required sutures if it wasn't scarring over. He examined it with an expression of curiosity and betrayal.

"I thought it would bleed more," he said. "Where's the artery?"

"Don't expect me to give you anatomy lessons."

Now he's serious.

"Can I examine your arm?"

"If it makes you happy."

I cleaned and bandaged the wounds.

He grinned, studying my work, the bulky dressing balling up at the palm and weaving between his fingers, making it difficult, if not impossible, to grip anything—especially a knife.

"I'm not blaming anybody," he said. "I'm meeting my troubles head on."

"It sure seems that way," I said.

"I love my kid. I want to be there for him, and I can't."

I didn't know what to say, so better to say nothing. "One of our most difficult duties as human beings is to listen to the voices of those who suffer," wrote Arthur Frank. "Listening is a hard but fundamentally moral act."

Outside the room, the voice from the patient who wanted narcotics rings down the corridor. "I'm in pain and nobody cares. I'm in fucking pain and does anybody care? Anybody?" Hospital security was escorting him out of the ER, and it felt wrong even though I'd explained the concerns from previous doctors and social workers about his substance use. He vehemently denied the overdoses documented in the record.

"I have no choice but to go back to heroin," he screamed. "It's on your head." His words, growing distant and small, burned like ice chips on the base of my neck. What if this isn't a threat? But he wasn't interested in other therapies or a pain clinic referral. I didn't doubt his pain. We disagreed on what counted as caring.

"Wow," said Mr. Atkins. "That's real."

"I'm sorry you had to hear that," I said, my breathing heavy and fast. Then he made a comment that knocked me over.

"This must be such a great job."

"Excuse me?"

"You know exactly what's going on. All the shit people do, the shit they must deal with."

I agreed with Mr. Atkins without entirely understanding what I agreed to. You can overthink such statements if you're not careful.

In his story "Gooseberries," Anton Chekhov wrote: "There ought to be behind the door of every happy, contented man some one standing with a hammer continually reminding him with a tap that there are unhappy people . . ."

"I *am* an expert in shit," I said, screeching my chair closer. "And there are many people in deep shit."

"I know."

"And they're still fighting. They haven't given up."

"I don't need a psychiatrist or medication."

"If we can get a better handle on the depression, perhaps your head will be in a better place to deal with your own shit."

"I need to keep my job and see my kid. It's simple."

"Is it that simple, Mr. Atkins?"

"If you want to hold onto me, do what you need to do."

"Mr. Atkins?"

"It's been tough," he said, laughing sadly. He raised his wrist, covered with a protective dressing, wearing an expression that blended betrayal and shame. How could he do such a thing? He'd never done anything like that before. He appeared frightened by this part of his self. But what scared him most was putting his already tenuous family situation in further jeopardy. Mr. Atkins pushed tears from his eyes. "I'm not crazy, doc."

"Of course not. Your excuse for not jumping off a bridge was fear of heights."

22
Unsafe Discharge

"Can we try to send Suzy home?" the nurse asks. It's an evening ER shift. Waiting patients line the hallways, including Suzy, who had been drinking at a local bar with friends and was later picked up by police walking home on the side of the road.

"Please," she says, clinging to my hand. "I don't belong here."

"Do you have a sober ride? Someone to look after you?"

"My boyfriend," she says, holding up her cell phone with its cracked screen as if it contained the answers to all her troubles. I ask if I could call and speak with him.

He's practiced in the conversation. He anticipates my questions. No, he's not drunk. And of course, he'll come, keep a close eye on her overnight. In the morning, he'll convince her to go back into rehab. An hour later, he arrives in the ER. Tall, stooped, haggard.

"Good luck," we say. She pushes her hand into his. So linked, they take the corner of the hallway toward the exit.

The next day Suzy is back in the ER, I come to discover. She was intoxicated again. And she's been beaten about the head and face. Knocked unconscious, jaw cracked in two places. According to the notes, she said her boyfriend did it—the responsible caregiver I had called to her bedside the night before.

23
Big Incision

The cardiac surgery team of fellows and residents was "rounding on me" the evening before my heart operation, and I wasn't comfortable being rounded on. Six months had passed since my near-syncopal episode while working a Labor Day ER shift, on the cusp of my forty-first birthday, and I was well into the imperfect practice of being a patient. "It must be hard being on the other side," a surgical resident said.

I was growing tired of this question. Some people were curious to hear what I had to say, but I sensed what this team of young doctors hid inside their inquiry was a need for solace, a shamanistic incantation that would protect them from my fate. Pneumonia, rapid atrial fibrillation, and a leaky mitral valve—all a surprise to someone who thought himself too busy to be sick. I could see them strain to pin a cause to my illness. But I'd been healthy. I watched my weight, exercised every day, and even flossed my teeth semi-regularly. My story refused to bend into a comforting cautionary tale. Their smiles wilted. They said goodbye and left the room.

Soon after, there was another knock on my door. A tall, casually dressed woman—the chaplain—apologized for disturbing me but wanted to check in. She knew I was a physician. From her somber calm, I could tell she knew of my diagnosis and the impending surgery.

"Are you scared?" she asked.

My wife sat wearily at my bedside. My son, five years old at the time, was back in Providence. "No," I lied.

She smiled stiffly, but there was a knowing warmth, too. She knew I was bullshitting her, and it was okay. She moved the conversation into another direction. "This experience will change the way you relate with patients, no?"

"I don't believe illness must be accompanied by great meaning," I told her. "Sometimes, a crummy heart valve is a crummy heart valve."

Genuine concern tightened her face.

My wife politely interjected. "It's been a long day."

The chaplain slipped her card upon the bedside stand.

"Patients often decide to talk after surgery."

"Thanks. I'll be okay."

"I'll ask the rabbi to visit?" she said before leaving.

I remembered my Long Island high holidays when I was younger. The spectacle, the sparkling dresses, the way a solemn occasion for reflection and religious observance turned into the Super Bowl of social status peacocking.

"If I need an ear," I said, struck by the chaplain's sincerity, "you'll be my first choice."

I didn't intend to be difficult, but being inside serious illness is different from talking about it. In her story "People

Like That Are the Only People Here," Lorrie Moore describes this translation challenge: "The trip and the story of the trip are always two different things. One cannot go to a place and speak of it, one cannot both see and say, not really."

For me, the ill person's mind earns its own logic, divines its own purposes. I resisted attempts to be buttoned inside a sentimental parable or hijacked by others as an example of what happens when you . . . what? . . . do shiftwork that makes a mockery of circadian rhythms? Work when sick? Rationalize symptoms that, in hindsight, point to a serious problem and not only a lack of sleep? Sure, I was a white coat in a hospital gown, but what I craved most was permission to be sick.

Serious illness had impacted my doctoring. I experienced firsthand the petty humiliations of being a patient—the barbaric stretchers, the ugly gowns, the theater of privacy afforded by curtains pretending to be walls. I joked with patients who can't find a comfortable position on the stretchers that if they didn't have back pain before, they'll have it when they leave. When patients and their families nervously waited for more information, I understood what sat behind their worry and checked in more often to let them know they hadn't been forgotten. I tried harder to arrange necessary services and secure follow-up appointments for the unfortunate patients without health insurance. Fighting illness is hard enough for patients without having to fight a broken healthcare system, too.

But this heightened empathy and compassion were balanced by other behaviors the chaplain might find less praiseworthy. I was intolerant of patients seeking doctor's notes for minor ailments to excuse them from work. I had a short fuse with rude patients and with families who lacked patience or possessed unreasonable expectations. I found myself sympathizing more with patients who didn't earn their fate, such as the young mother with ovarian or breast cancer, than those like the middle-aged man who drank alcohol daily who had fallen down his basement stairs.

The further I traveled into my illness, I discovered fewer recognizable roads for my type of journey. Months after first becoming ill—and countless failed attempts at electrical cardioversion—it became evident that my problems weren't going away and my leaky mitral valve needed repair or replacement. Suddenly, I became someone in need of a cardiac surgeon. Friends and colleagues at a prestigious medical center immediately recommended Dr. A, a humanist with excellent hands. My cardiologist insisted on a famous heart surgeon (FHS) in the department at the same institution. One of my closest friends, a cardiac surgeon at a distant medical center, counseled me about the FHS, his accolades and skills, as well as his notorious personality. He shared stories from others who had endured the FHS's wrath as a rite of passage to their illustrious careers.

"That shouldn't concern you," my buddy said. "You'll be under anesthesia."

My wife and I arranged to meet these two giants on the same day. That morning, we entered Dr. A's world. He came out into the waiting room to greet us. His pressed white coat was devoid of the ink and coffee stains that marked mine;

the knot of his silk tie a work of art. He led us into his office, warmed with dark wood and soft chairs. His carefully chosen words were crafted into lucid paragraphs, tailored to fit my ears and those of my non-medical wife. His physical examination matched that of any uber-internist. By the end of the hour, I wanted him as my surgeon, friend, mentor, and life coach.

Afterward, my wife and I lunched ravenously in the hospital cafeteria. Our consultation with the FHS awaited us, but it was only a formality. We had Dr. A in our back pocket.

An administrative assistant took us through a maze of cubicles to get to the FHS's office, where he acknowledged us from behind his desk. The FHS donned a navy blazer over scrubs and expensive-looking leather shoes. He gave the impression that he was squeezing us into his schedule, and thus, we shouldn't bother with small talk about my symptoms. He offered me a matter-of-fact look—he rarely acknowledged my wife—raised my thick medical chart as if it explained everything, and dropped it onto the desk. The thump itself, I could only guess, served as a verdict. "You need an operation," he said. "Questions?"

Was he kidding? He must be kidding. He wasn't joking. I heard my wife whimpering for Dr. A.

I felt part of a Monty Python skit. An anesthesiologist would soon appear, the surgical team would hop out from the cubicles, and they'd open my chest and do the plumbing work on my heart right here, right now, on his immense desk.

I tried to penetrate the FHS's brazen exterior, find warmth behind his steely blue eyes. He discounted my questions about stroke complications from the bypass pump. "You're young." I asked about the long-term success rate of valve repairs, if my valve could be saved. "We don't have long-term data. But you're young." I asked about his work doing mitral valve surgery with a small chest wall incision instead of the median sternotomy, citing studies in the surgical literature by his team. I confessed that the possibility of less pain and faster recovery appealed to me. The FHS quickly killed that surgical option. "You need a maze, too," he said, alluding to a procedure where the surgeon creates a maze pattern of scar tissue in the upper chamber of the heart to block the abnormal impulses from atrial fibrillation.

"Atrial fib and the heart valve," he said. "You're looking at a big incision."

I was transported back to the intimidating surgeons at medical school and during my residency. Only I was an attending now. I was a patient.

"We had a consultation with Dr. A this morning," I said.

He nodded respectfully, then gave me a look that was scalpel sharp. "Remember this," he said. "Your problem is nothing special. I did two of you this morning."

On the way out, we were left to negotiate the maze of cubicles on our own. Once beyond the office doors, I felt relieved and disoriented, as if we'd just stepped off a gravity-defying amusement ride. My wife and I slowly walked the corridor, passed the framed paintings of famous heart surgeons casting their icy stares. We stopped, faced each other. "He's our guy," we declared at the same time.

What? The decision defied rational explanation. Just a few hours earlier, we had invested our confidence, thoroughly and without reservation, in the empathic and talented Dr. A. But did I need empathy, someone to hold my hand? I reconsidered Dr. A's responsible and cautious detailing of the surgery, his honest admission that the valve might be too damaged for repair. That meant replacement, and possibly lifelong anticoagulation. The FHS didn't express such gravity. He seemed bored with my heart problem, even annoyed by it. Did he routinely inform patients that their problems weren't special? Or was he savvy to the workings of the physician-patient's mind, and his brusqueness functioned as a communication strategy?

Each time I tell this story, I'm greeted with genuine shock from students and colleagues who can't believe I passed over the ideal embodiment of a surgeon in favor of someone who couldn't be summed up as easily. They don't expect this detour, this upending of their expectations. What's more, I detect slight discomfort from them, a defensiveness, unsure of this story's moral takeaway. Surely, I'm not saying we shouldn't make time to be an empathic and articulate communicator. If there is a moral to this story, it's be careful of the appetite you bring to stories. From the moment I set eyes on the FHS, this complicated character, I knew what type of surgeon I was hungry for—an accomplished, hard-driving, and unsentimental adversary.

How could I explain this reasoning to the big-hearted hospital chaplain or the nervous surgical team who brought their respective expectations to my story? My body might have failed me. But my story would have disappointed them.

Long after the chaplain left my room and my wife went home to our son, there was a soft tap on my door. A medical student in a short white coat asked if he could do a medical history and physical examination. Sleep and worry tugged on my sleeve, but I waved him in.

"You're a doctor?" he said after finishing the perfunctory questions and briefly running through the exam. I smiled. "Does it feel strange?" he asked, nodding to my place on the bed.

"A little," I said.

"Are you scared?"

I don't know whether it was his lack of responsibility for me or his innocent and distressed look when asking these questions, but somehow this kid had upended my defenses.

"A lot," I said.

Fear hit me hard. I sat up higher, as straight as I could. I could be glib with the chaplain because I knew she'd see through it. But he was licking his lips. He was more than interested in what I had to say. He looked thirsty for it.

"Be wary of scripts," I said. "Patients shouldn't feel miscast in their illness." The student's gaze didn't waver. "You did a good job. Doctors are complicated patients."

The morning of my heart surgery, after a nurse's aide nearly broke an electric razor shaving my chest hair, I lay under a sheet in pre-op, more naked than I'd ever thought possible. The FHS entered. We shook hands for the first time since our meeting several months before. He appeared well rested, freshly showered. He kept tapping my chart as if he couldn't wait to start. How can I describe my emotions? My fear was swept up inside his energy, his confidence, his focus. So much was happening that resisted making any sense. A sedative started swimming through the IV. I didn't feel calm. My body asserted itself, assumed a weightless density and cocky buzz, and I welcomed its invitation to retreat into it.

"See you inside," the FHS said.

Those words floated around my fuzzy head. Did he mean inside the operating room, or inside my chest? He was about to turn away but stopped. "What are we doing again?"

Was he serious?

"Mitral valve. Maze."

"That's right." He delicately drew a straight line with his index finger over my chest.

"Big incision," he said, and winked.

When the FHS rounded on me in the cardiac surgery ICU the day after the surgery and told me he expected me to get out of bed and into a chair, I'd already done that. I loved the surprise in his face when, a day or two later, he learned I was already walking around the corridor. I was discharged from the hospital earlier than expected, and I took pleasure in the FHS's discomfort with this plan. They had pulled the catheter from neck and the tube from my chest. The cardiac rehab experts gave me the green light. But it wasn't a smart move. As much as I craved being home, I lost my adversary. Focusing on upending the FHS's expectations was a major force of motivation and distraction. Once home, I couldn't pretend my sternum hadn't been cracked open, that breathing hurt, coughing hurt like hell, and somehow I had to get back to seeing ER patients in a month. The surgery ended with recovery, but the resolution of illness, and my development as a patient, dragged on.

This particular story, however, has an ending. Six weeks later, at the end of my follow-up appointment, I quickly told the FHS how grateful I was for his team's care, especially all the nurses and therapists. He laid his hand lightly and ever so briefly on my shoulder, then left to see his next patient.

24
To Err Is to Be a Physician

An early morning, unexpected call at home from an ER colleague: "Remember Mr. Mull? You saw him yesterday?"

My legs began to wobble. In emergency medicine, "remember that patient" is usually the opening line to terrible news.

"He came back in the middle of the night," he said.

My coffee mug, half empty, grew heavy in my hand.

"The medics were doing CPR."

A long silence.

"He didn't make it."

My body went numb. I lowered myself slowly into a kitchen chair.

What? What happened?

I cared for Mr. Mull, a lovely man in his mid-fifties, most of the shift. He came to the ER with chest pain. No, shoulder pain, he then said, squeezing his left shoulder. No, chest pain. Both symptoms raise concern for a possible heart attack or unstable angina. His recently diagnosed mild diabetes was also a risk factor for coronary artery disease. But his chest pain was sharp. It hurt when he twisted and moved. He jumped off the stretcher and pushed my hands away when I palpated his chest, shoulder, and upper back. Such alarming sensitivity pointed to a muscular or bony source of the pain, or maybe herpes zoster, though I couldn't find a rash.

What did I miss?

My suspicion for a heart problem was very low, but given his age, the loose feel of his story, and the fact that diabetes can present with atypical heart attack symptoms, I pursued a standard chest pain workup, including an EKG, chest X-ray, and cardiac markers for a heart attack. The results reassuring, I called Mr. Mull's primary care physician, who told me Mr. Mull suffered from chronic pain, for which he was prescribed opioids. Mr. Mull's doctor asked if I thought anything serious was going on—shorthand for worrisome causes of chest pain such as a heart attack, a blood clot in the lung, a dissection of the aorta, a collapsed lung, pneumonia. If not, he'd follow up with Mr. Mull first thing in the morning. I had a low threshold for admitting patients with chest pain to the hospital, I told him, and yet I was comfortable discharging him home.

To my surprise, to everyone's surprise, the autopsy couldn't find a definitive cause for his death. Over twenty years later, this lack of evidence sits uneasily because something in his body went terribly and unexpectedly wrong.

I met the family for the first and only time after the autopsy results were released, during which I found myself saying words that trouble me to this day. I walked them through each step in my decision-making process. Mr. Mull's son, a man in his twenties, asked if I'd have done anything differently given what I know now. I felt a dry ball in the back of the throat. "Not a thing," I said, fighting back the tears. "I'd do everything exactly the same."

What a crazy thing to say, especially when a patient—and more importantly, a husband and a father—had died. An identifiable cause of death would have given me something to learn from, to take with me, to ensure that it would never happen again.

I was a young but experienced attending at the time. I ruminated about patients after my shift was over. When trying to sleep, I was hounded by diagnoses I should have considered or tests I might have ordered or documentation that could have demonstrated my reasoning in greater detail. And yet, the evening before, I never second-guessed my care for Mr. Mull.

Most so-called experts are confident, even overconfident, in their decisions. Physicians are no exception. The calibration between diagnostic accuracy and a physician's confidence in that accuracy doesn't always line up. In one study, physicians were given easy and hard case vignettes and offered opportunities to request more resources, information, or input from others at various stages along the decision-making process. Researchers found the difficult cases resulted in a decline in diagnostic accuracy but not a proportionate drop-off in confidence.

But it makes sense. If we believe we're right, it's hard to recognize any need for more information. This study highlights a central challenge of being wrong, which Kathryn Schulz described so elegantly in her book *Being Wrong*.

There's a difference between being wrong and feeling wrong, she wrote. When you're in the moment, being wrong feels a lot like being right.

In medicine, we're taught that the more evidence we accumulate and the more thoroughly and objectively we evaluate it, the more accurate our diagnosis or decision-making will be. And if we make a mistake, well, we didn't have enough evidence, or we interpreted it wrong. But when you're in the decision-making moment, how do we know the evidence you've accumulated is enough evidence?

Experts for the plaintiff in my case said I didn't gather enough evidence. A part of me agrees. For years I've been haunted by that vital, elusive golden nugget.

What we believe to be evidence-based knowledge is often constructed out of probability and likelihood, a cloud of data points that, taken together, allow us to draw reliable judgments about a population as a whole. But a single patient can fall through the cloud. Medicine doesn't know what to do with a single case. If it results in a good outcome, we shrug and say one case counts as an anecdote; more research needs to be done. However, tragedies need an explanation, and sweeping conclusions are often drawn even if the connection to the outcome is unclear.

Mr. Mull's covering doctor told me she would have sent him home, too. Others said I should have admitted Mr. Mull to the hospital overnight. The insistent voices in my head agreed with this group, who couldn't debate otherwise in hindsight. Though, if blinded to the outcome, I'd likely make the same decision given the same situation.

The narrative I desperately needed was unavailable to me, one that disentangled unfortunate outcomes and possible error from the specter of malpractice, whose purpose was insight, not blame, and one that made room for us to sink into uncertainty, sympathy, sorrow, and apology.

Nancy Berlinger has described medical harm in the context of broken stories, resulting in a communication breakdown between patients/families and physicians/healthcare institutions and a fragmenting of trust. When the flow of information stops or reduces to a trickle, families may suspect the healthcare team and the hospital are hiding something even if they hadn't earlier. Broken stories become sources of further harm. I experienced and witnessed the spiritual brokenness she describes, the suffering felt by providers, patients, and families resulting from a rupture in the mutual expectation that the physician will do no harm.

I felt accountable for their tragedy. But hospital legal council cautioned me to avoid any language of apology, such as "I'm sorry." An apology is a human expression of remorse for another's pain. But an apology at this time, in this context, could be used by the plaintiff's lawyer as an admittance of fault. I wasn't prepared for the friction produced by the emotions I wanted to express and the guarded line of defense I was expected to uphold. My only genuine human connection with this tragedy was the afternoon I sat with the family, answering their questions, sharing tears, and bearing the full force of their loss and my role in it.

To be a physician is to be tormented by the inevitability of poor outcomes. The word "error" has origins in the

Latin *errare*, meaning "to roam" or "to wander." It's easier to rationalize the possibility of error, especially in emergency medicine, which often involves diagnosing high-risk, low-probability conditions under demanding conditions where ambiguity and uncertainty rule. Once it happens, however, distinguishing fallibility from inevitability can leave you feeling panicked, chased by disgrace and doubt, an outcast from previous conceptions of yourself as a good doctor.

In 1999, the Institute of Medicine (IOM) report *To Err Is Human* . . . launched the patient safety movement in the United States with the news that 44,000 to 98,000 hospitalized patients die each year because of medical error. From their definition of error, described as "either a failure of a planned action to be completed as intended or the use of the wrong plan to achieve an aim," any untoward outcome could be interpreted as medical error. This overly broad definition muddies the relationship between poor outcomes and medical error.

Dr. Hardeep Singh and colleagues have developed a different paradigm, one of missed opportunities, which acknowledges the complexity of the diagnostic process, that poor outcomes often result from processes done well and a wrong diagnosis might not have been wrong at that moment in time. Unless we examine these moments with an eye on the contingent conditions and the available information at the moment, the focus on not missing anything may further compromise patient safety by promoting overtesting, with its own concomitant risks in addition to driving up healthcare costs. For the longest time afterward, I lost all trust in my ability and my instincts. I overtested and admitted patients to the hospital I might have previously sent home.

If mastery exists in medical practice, it's refining the process of interrogating what we know and why we think we know it. I'll never forget the son's response to the inconclusive autopsy results: So they're saying my father died a healthy man? When a patient dies, it doesn't matter if it's the result of an error or a missed opportunity; it's almost impossible to argue to others or convince yourself that the decisions you made were the right ones.

The IOM report illuminated this central and yet unresolvable tension in its title: *To Err Is Human* . . . If to err is human, and physicians are human, shouldn't there exist a degree of tolerance for physicians who make mistakes or find themselves party to a tragic outcome?

At night, I'd apologize to Mr. Mull and his family and ask for their forgiveness, a habit that continued long after the case was settled. Gradually, I found my way out of the shame, regret, and sadness. I shed enough self-doubt to discover myself as an ER doc who was a bit dented and bruised but otherwise salvageable and in decent working order. The words "remember that patient" were the opening lines to my darkest fears and later became the operating instructions for moving forward. Mr. Mull is forever part of my story as an emergency physician. The narrative of emergency medicine never stops asking for more. There's always another patient to see, another person depending on me, two imperfect humans straining to connect under imperfect circumstances.

25
When Sensitivity Is a Liability

You find a spot in the shadows of the ER. A nurse has turned off a bank of overhead lamps, creating a twilight that's anything but peaceful. You fidget with the stethoscope pocketed in the white coat you never wear, listening to your patient's father and aunt as they stand vigil over the stretcher. You're all waiting for the young man to die a second time.

"I shouldn't have let him take the Chevy," says the father, a stooped refrigerator of a man wearing work boots, a Patriots sweatshirt, and a limp.

"He just got out of rehab," says the aunt, her face a mystery of lines—too much sun, too much smoking, too much worry. "This shouldn't happen."

The aunt shoots you a look, as if she expects you, an ER doc, to be some expert on should. But should you be standing a full two strides away from him? A pulse should trigger a celebration, especially when the patient is young and dying. Instead, you're begging his heart to quit and rethinking the decision to put on the white coat. It makes promises it can't deliver.

You shared certain details with the father and aunt. Friends found him in the pickup with a needle in his arm.

Pulseless. Not breathing. Probably not breathing for a while. They called 911. EMS said he was gray and cool, his skin mottled. EMS worked themselves into a sweat for a half-hour on the scene. Naloxone. Chest compressions. Breathing tube. Epinephrine.

Other details you withheld. EMS said the friends were barely coherent. He was parked outside a drug house, a notorious triple-decker, covered in vomit and blood from a tongue bite. At least a half-hour had gone by before someone checked on him and called 911. The initial cardiac rhythm was asystole, an ominous state of electrical quiet that resisted all EMS interventions. And when they rushed him in, pounding on his chest, you thought about calling the code.

"Why did I give him the keys?" says the father.

"You showed trust," says the aunt.

"Yeah, right. I didn't want to knock heads on his first day home."

Five minutes without oxygen starts the clock on permanent brain damage. Half an hour had passed before 911 was even called, so total downtime was pushing an hour. A dismal prognosis. But this is your third overdose that evening. You felt this urge, more like a pressure, to do something. He's young. He's healthy. A lifetime awaits. You hear your voice order another round of epinephrine, a few more minutes of CPR. But soon after, when the nurse yells, "I got a pulse," a part of you begins to sink. Why make the effort if success just means prolonging a family's pain?

"Does he have to be so stubborn?" the father says, blowing his nose, pushing the empty chair away. You scour the entire ER for the two chairs that they don't sit in. The aunt nods thanks. The father says, "I want my son back and you give me a chair?"

There's no logic to your caring. The brain CT showed changes commonly seen in patients with severe anoxic brain injury, which only confirmed your fears. Without the ventilator to breathe for him and the medications to support his blood pressure, he'd die. "He wouldn't have wanted this," his father says through angry tears, gesturing at the ventilator and the IV drips. "No more," the father says, and requests that we change his son's goals of care to comfort measures only.

Earlier this shift, you used naloxone to reverse overdoses in two other patients. One of them, a middle-aged woman, had OD'd that morning and almost succeeded again later that evening. Yet you didn't feel joy. Your emotions were slippery. Sorrow and resignation. Compassion and blame. Saving them from death is easier than saving them from themselves, you thought, but the latter is impossible unless you first save them from death and save them from death again.

"He's in the Lord's hands," the aunt says.

The father shrugs. "The Lord wasn't doing a bang-up job keeping an eye on him up to now."

Some people treat their body like a temple. Others treat it like a chemistry set. Understanding motives, even your own, is always tricky. Judgment seeps into the cracks. The bottom line is you can't truly understand the horror of a drug-hijacked brain—the pain, the hopelessness, the unbearable need for escape. You turn off the heart monitor so they won't hear death take him. They fill that silence with memories, which only conjure him back to life. Now the gray body in cardiac arrest is an ex-boyfriend of his old high school flame and the father of a boy in kindergarten—the one thing they did right together—who made his face light up.

You can't leave the patient and the family after your shift is over. That's your fingerprints on their grief.

"He stuck it out, finished rehab," says the father, not realizing what you know: that the body's tolerance for narcotics goes down in rehab. People in recovery become more sensitive to the drug, and this sensitivity can kill them should they relapse. You feel the cruel irony that sensitivity is a liability. You want to make things right, only it's too late for that. So you stand in the room, listening to their troubles—once again, you realize, providing the wrong help at the wrong time for the wrong reasons.

26

Why Won't My Patient Act Like a Jerk?

I'm avoiding Mr. G's room. I shouldn't have read the ER notes from the other hospital, where this middle-aged man raised a stink about the wait. What type of person calls the triage nurse a bitch? From the timestamps on the electronic medical record notes, he stormed from that ER and drove his abdominal pain, vomiting, diarrhea, and discontent directly across town to us.

I'm reminded of this oft-quoted aphorism from Sir William Osler: "The good physician treats the disease; the great physician treats the patient who has the disease." It's cited by medical educators as an invocation never to forget the humanistic heart at the center of clinical care. But what if the patient is a jerk?

That I haven't met Mr. G, only read briefly about him, doesn't stop these ugly feelings from surfacing. I dart to the bathroom. Scrub my face. Force a wide smile into the mirror. I can't decide whether vigorous soaping and working my happy muscles serve as therapy or procrastination. Regardless, I must dig in and care for him.

To compensate for this judgment, to hedge against letting my feelings leak through, I introduce myself in an overly cheerful tone: "Good evening, Mr. G! How can I help you?"

I brace for the lashing tongue.

"Hi doc," he says.

His manner is disarmingly friendly. There's no rant about the scene at the other ER or the wait in ours. He describes his daughter's twenty-four-hour gastrointestinal bug that jumped to his wife, who spent a day racing between bed and bathroom. And now it's his turn. Only less vomiting and more diarrhea, body aches, and awful abdominal cramps. And it's day three.

"What do you think? A viral thing?"

Who is this polite guy? Where's the insulting brute I had expected? I scroll through the computer, believing I've confused him with another patient. But it's him. My opinions about Mr. G may feel justified and real, even though I built an opinion of this person after breezing through a few short notes, without ever meeting him. That the medical record contains objective findings—blood work or radiographic imaging or operative notes—can create an impression that all notes are equally objective when many are first-person narratives written from a single health provider's point of view. It's one side of the story, possibly shaded with biases and emotions.

Then my eyes fix on an old note that mentions a substance use problem. Narcotics. I consider his body aches, vomiting, diarrhea, and abdominal cramps. These are symptoms of opioid withdrawal. Intense craving for narcotics and altered neurochemistry could explain his behavior at the other ER, too. But he denies substance use.

Do I believe what my patient is telling me? Doubt is a particularly uncomfortable form of uncertainty, especially when a person's integrity is under question and that person is a patient. When a physician doesn't fully trust a patient, caring can feel like a chore. I take a swig of coffee and head back to his room.

I must ask Mr. G without signaling my suspicion. Understandably, patients don't take kindly to such lines of inquiry. And they haven't come down off a rage-filled incident at another ER. I frame my query from the perspective of his pain and comfort. If he's using opioids, I'll have to adjust my pain strategy accordingly. If he's in withdrawal, my treatment approach to quell his symptoms will change.

He calmly describes the terrible car accident that left him with a fractured femur, pelvis, and lumbar spine. Then, there's the ordeal that put him back together, the surgeries, the painful rehab, his dependence on narcotics. However, that was many years ago. The medication list in our medical records is an old one.

Besides, the cardinal features of withdrawal are absent. Heart isn't racing. Hair on his arms isn't standing up. Pupils aren't the size of sunflowers. But sadly, I can reason together details in any number of ways to support the impression that I've already arrived at.

He suspects the vomiting yanked his chronically bad back. His exam is consistent with a muscle spasm. I suggest medications for his vomiting, muscle relaxants, and intravenous fluids. I wait for him to call out his pain and to insist on something stronger.

But he says: "Sounds good, doc."

Really? I think. Because this encounter doesn't feel good to me. When tossed into the waters between belief and doubt, it's hard to reach either shore.

An hour passes, then two. He says the symptoms have eased off a little, but he's not better. I order more medications. "Sounds good, doc," he says, again. During some playful banter, I can't help but wonder when the real Mr. G will roar to the surface. As I'm leaving his room, he freezes me. "One more thing . . ."

Here's the doorknob moment, I thought, when the patient drops a crucial piece of information that's often shameful or difficult right when the provider is about to leave the room. This new revelation often reboots the encounter. Sometimes, it's a dreaded, nonchalant request for narcotic medications. But at this moment, halting before the half-drawn curtain, I want Mr. G to demand Dilaudid or morphine. I desperately need him to act out. By becoming the insulting guy at the other ER, he can validate my assumptions about him that I can't shake. If he doesn't, it exposes a dark, hollow in me I'd rather not see.

"Can I get more fluid through the IV," he says. "I feel dehydrated."

"Sure," I say. My self-image resembles the crinkled IV bag that hangs empty on a pole at the head of his stretcher. "I'll get another liter up right away." I turn to leave.

"Doc?" He takes a long pause, then offers his hand. "Thanks for treating me like a human being."

My return handshake is just as firm, only it's an apology for making quick judgments and using seeming kindness to disguise them.

His abdominal pain persists. I try to convince myself that the tenderness in his lower right belly wasn't there before. The truth is, I had created a story about him, and it shaped, in part, how I processed and interpreted objective findings. Symptoms of appendicitis can mimic opiate withdrawal and gastroenteritis. The possibility that I've been sitting on appendicitis makes me sick. It changes the polarity of the encounter. If confirmed, the delay becomes an inexcusable medical error and his rude behavior, seen through the lens of a serious diagnosis, gets recast as a missed cry for help.

The CT scan—the "donut of truth" to doctors—reveals no clear explanation for his symptoms. Never before have I been this grateful for uncertainty. Mr. G is soon sipping apple juice and nibbling on crackers. A comfort has developed between us, and I decide to quiz him a little about the incident at the other ER.

His body stiffens. "They didn't care," he says.

I remind him about the medication list in his medical record, the old notes. I wonder aloud if the triage nurse, too, jumped to conclusions about substance use. His complaining and cursing probably didn't help matters. I explain the triage nurse's demanding job. On nights when the hospital is full and admitted patients stop up the ER, the waiting room can heat into a cauldron of frustration. The human heart isn't designed to withstand the constant assaults that triage nurses absorb.

"I hate coming to the ER," he says. "I don't get sick. The diarrhea was bad. Real bad."

I mention what I read in his record, what he had yelled.

"I said that?" He looks around.

I nod. "It seems that way."

"I was running to the toilet. I mean running. For hours. Once I didn't make it, if you get what I mean. I had to toss my underwear. And I'm told there are sick patients ahead of me?" His voice rises. "Really?" He takes a breath and holds it.

He appears more embarrassed by the words he shouted than the diarrhea. "Can I ask a favor?"

"You can ask."

"Clarify things. I'm not that guy."

"I'll write that you're pleasant and cooperative."

"And the med list," he says. "I don't take narcotics."

I'm discharging Mr. G, and a critical part of his treatment is just beginning—tending to his medical record. Mr. G is that guy, but he's also the gentleman sitting on the edge of the stretcher. I frequently meet patients on the computer screen, through their medical record, before I ever shake their hands. Being familiar with their medical backstory can bring comfort to patients. But taking shortcuts is risky business. The medical record is a scrapbook of test results and the reports of others. The reader creates an impression of truth. Now caring for Mr. G means making him knowable to the next physician or nurse who reads about him. And in the process, making sure I do better by the next Mr. G.

27
Wheelchair

After midnight, leaving an evening shift, I stumbled on a hospital wheelchair parked on the second floor of the parking garage. It was too small for the space, appeared exposed and lost in the vast emptiness. But someone situated it dutifully between the lines, as if grateful for explicit rules and guidance about what's expected of them. I imagined the person who put it there, the family or friend they helped transfer from the wheelchair into the car, the fleeting sense of control from aligning it just so. Or, maybe the wheelchair was a subtle and startling effort by someone to have their troubles recognized. Or, it could all be a joke. Each possibility is incomplete, unpolished, and strangely human. It is all spawned from a single wheelchair discovered in an unexpected place where it shouldn't belong—yet somehow it does.

III
Possibility

The temptation towards resolution, towards wrapping
up the package, seems to me a terrible trap. Why not
be more honest with the moment? The most authentic
endings are the ones which are already revolving
towards another beginning.

—Sam Shepard

28
Caring for the Caregiver

Mrs. G has been in the ER for hours. An exhaustive workup hasn't revealed a serious cause for her weakness, the reason her daughter Maureen brought her in. I explain that Mrs. G appears dehydrated and, after the rest of the intravenous fluids runs in, she can probably go home. Mrs. G's eyes light up while her daughter's go blank. I sense that Maureen expected, maybe even hoped, that her mother would need to stay in the hospital, even just for the night.

Maureen had given me a brick of paperwork neatly fastened with a black metal binder clip inside a worn manila envelope. It chronicles what has become of Mrs. G's life—enduring the unforgiving fates of congestive heart failure, diabetes, high blood pressure, mild kidney failure, osteoporosis, depression, and early dementia. It also details her last hospital admission for pneumonia, an extended stay that left her with an open ulcer on the skin over her tailbone that, months later, still hasn't healed. Maureen was worried that another bout of pneumonia was brewing.

"I'd like to see your mom drink something," I tell Maureen, then catch myself. I was disrespecting Mrs. G by talking around her and directing the conversation to her daughter. After decades of doctoring, I should know better. That an older patient sits in silence doesn't mean she hasn't a strong voice in her care; that she carries a diagnosis of dementia doesn't necessarily imply she can't comprehend what I'm saying. Even if her understanding is incomplete, respect demands that I include her as much as possible; she's the focus of our conversation.

"Can you try to drink something?" I ask Mrs. G, pointing to a Styrofoam cup half-filled with ice and water.

Maureen folds a sheet and slips it behind her mother's back as a pillow. "Drink up," she says. "Did you hear what the doctor said?"

"What?"

"You have to drink more."

Maureen sighs, then laments her mother's hearing troubles.

I ask if one ear works better than the other.

Maureen points to her mother's left ear. As she steps aside so I can lean closer, she mentions how her mother's hearing can be very fickle. Sometimes she hears you just fine. Depends on what you're saying to her.

Her mother rolls her eyes. "She's stubborn," Maureen says, smiling. "I try everything to get her to drink. Water. Tea. Juice."

"Who helps care for her?" I ask.

"It's me," she says with a stiff smile.

Maureen alludes to her brothers and sisters, how they don't understand how hard it is, and they're not around much to find out.

Her face can no longer disguise the strain. I soon realize the most acutely distressed person in the exam room isn't Mrs. G but her daughter, her caregiver.

Caregivers are typically family members responsible for looking after the daily needs of someone, or multiple people, who are frail, sick, or disabled. Caregiving tasks can be all-consuming. They include feeding, dressing, grooming, assisting with toiletry, bathing, shopping, cooking, housekeeping, and doing laundry. The work can extend to arranging transportation, handling financial matters, and scheduling doctor visits. They juggle a menu of medications; a third of older adults take five or more every day.

Caregivers often do their noble work in the shadows even though a large national survey has revealed that one in five Americans serve as unpaid caregivers, and another 17 percent expect to become caregivers in the two years after the survey. Not surprisingly, studies show that close to 70 percent of caregivers are women.

Maureen is concerned the slight fever earlier in the day points to an infection we're not seeing yet. "Wouldn't it be safer to keep her in the hospital?" she asks. Moving her mother to and from the car is a chore. She doesn't want to get home only to have to bring her back to the hospital.

I find myself looking differently at Mrs. G's daughter. Is she hoping to leverage her mother's symptoms for a break, a soft version of what has been called "granny dumping"? I was introduced to that concept during the first Thanksgiving of my emergency medicine residency. Families would drop off their older relatives at the ER with a packed bag and nebulous complaints and then take off, expecting the hospital to care for them. Other judgment-filled euphemisms include "positive taillight sign" and "packed suitcase syndrome." This phenomenon happens in other countries as well.

I would be infuriated with these families, especially when they didn't stick around to talk to the physicians. But, with experience, I have learned this problem is more nuanced, often the end product of social conditions and systems that fail to provide enough resources for caregivers who often face daunting tasks. A University of Michigan study showed that Medicare patients who are looked after by caregivers who score high for fatigue and low for health status and depression incur higher healthcare costs, including more ER visits. Another study found that dementia patients with caregivers suffering from symptoms of depression are twice as likely to visit the ER than persons whose caregivers aren't depressed. Caregiver obligations are equivalent to unpaid full-time jobs that include overnights and weekends. Could anyone blame them for seeking a breather?

Providing critical support for others can be a source of burnout—especially when caregivers don't get the help they need, try to handle too much, or take on things they aren't capable of. Even when undertaken from a wellspring of generosity and love, caregiving can produce physical, emotional, and psychological exhaustion. The psychological distress and physical demands associated with caregiving are reflected in a disturbing range of biological responses, from slower wound healing to elevated blood pressure and an impaired immune response, resulting in an overall increase in caregiver mortality. Over 20 percent of caregivers in many states rate their own health as fair or poor. When caregivers do carve out time for themselves, they are inclined to feel guilty about it, resulting in a paradoxical worsening of their burnout. And yet, we don't expend much energy probing the caregiver's experience, discussing the burdens of such work, and recognizing the challenges they face.

It's embarrassing to admit this, but it wasn't until Maureen shared what worried her about taking her mother home that I noticed how worn she looked. Her uncombed hair, loose sweatshirt, baggy sweatpants, and Crocs without socks; the slope of her sagging shoulders, the heaviness behind her dark eyes, the bravery in her quivering smile.

Caregivers, I've learned, make uneasy patients when their bodies cry for attention. So focused on someone else's needs, they can't prioritize their own. I once cared for a middle-aged woman with signs of a heart attack, including a worrisome EKG. She refused to stay in the hospital for further evaluation because she cared for her mother with dementia. Unless she cared for herself, I said, she can't care for others who depend on her. "Let me care for you so you can care for your mom?" I begged. Ultimately, she apologized, as if she was letting me down, and left anyway.

I turn to address both Mrs. G and Maureen. "I'd like to consult a social worker," I say.

There are so many situations such as this one where the social worker quickly becomes the most indispensable member of the treatment team. Social workers are trained to assess a patient's needs as well as caregiver's roles, capacities, vulnerabilities, and strengths in a nonjudgmental manner. I've learned so much from their ability to parse through complex situations using a deep knowledge of human psychology, family dynamics, bureaucratic red tape, health insurance fine print, and local home and community services. They dive into the messiness of life and somehow conjure possible solutions with sensitivity, savvy, and spunk. For the less skilled in this type of inquiry—such as myself—there are valuable guides for busy families and busy health professionals, such as the resources available in the Next Step in Care program produced by the United Hospital Fund.

A vital part of Mrs. G's treatment includes finding opportunities to lighten Maureen's load. But Maureen quickly refuses. She has everything under control, she says, adding that they can't afford extra services.

I'm not surprised. An estimated 14.7 million older adults receive assistance with daily activities from spouses and family caregivers. Unfortunately, only one-quarter of caregivers take advantage of supportive services, possibly because they may not perceive themselves as caregivers, a term with professional connotations. They're wives and husbands, sons and daughters, nieces and nephews, parents and friends. They're also vital partners to the healthcare ecosystem, a treasure trove of information and insight when the patient has trouble communicating with the medical staff or appear to be withholding or dismissing problematic aspects of the story.

The critical role of caregivers became achingly evident when COVID-19 struck, and many hospitals, to safeguard the threat of infection, didn't permit visitors such as family. When patients have dementia, or are confused or lethargic because of a medical issue, getting a clear idea of a patient's story can be challenging. Sometimes, a note appears in the medical record with the name and number of a caregiver contact who is nervously waiting. Other times, we chase phone numbers and leave unanswered messages, or find bothered family members or machine voices that a number is no longer in service.

Without Maureen's presence, my care of Mrs. G would be limited. For all the information in the medical record, I'd lack context, the interpretive window into the history and personality of Mrs. G. Looking back, I can't say how this encounter would unfold under the constraints of COVID-19. Over the phone, I doubt I'd have picked up on Maureen's strain without the visual cues. I believe Maureen would be eagerly waiting for my call. But I can also imagine a scenario where Maureen sounds a tad grumpy when I wake her, having collapsed into desperately needed sleep.

Sometimes, caring for patients requires that we reach into the shadows and shine a light on their caregivers. At the very least we can recognize that caregiving is difficult and that should they seek help or hint for a break, it isn't a sign of weakness or failure.

Maureen doesn't want to discuss possible remedies to her caregiving challenges. I wonder about her stiff resolve, whether our offer of assistance also exposes her to judgment. Her siblings might consider her need for outside help to be a failure on her part.

So I do what I can. I make a point of saying she is doing a great job with her mother. I highlight the pressure sore in her mother's lower back. It is clean and healing, at least as well as those things heal. "That's a tough wound to care for," I say. "Really tough."

"It is," she says. "Thank you for saying that."

29
Oktoberfest

"Really?" I say to one of our regular alcohol users. "It's 10 a.m."

"You don't understand, doc. It's Oktoberfest."

"No."

"It is."

"I'm saying that's not a good excuse."

He waves me off. "You don't know what you're talking about."

"For you, every day is Oktoberfest. And when every day is Oktoberfest, no day is Oktoberfest."

His face twists into many shapes as he thinks on this. A big smile lights up, as if I understand him perfectly, or misunderstood him imperfectly, or maybe he appreciates my attempt at humor because the lamest joke is an invitation to share a moment.

30
Dr. Douchebag

"We're going to take good care of you," I reassure Mr. Blunt. EMS said two bullets. The trauma team examining him from head to toe found the wound in the right thigh, but nothing in the right flank, the other possible site.

"And you are?" Mr. Blunt says.

I'd already introduced myself, but he's really after my position in the hierarchy. "I'm one of the doctors in charge," I say.

"Good." He sighs. "Call my cousin."

"First things first," I say, telling him we need to make sure there isn't a life-threatening injury that requires immediate attention. After we're done with this part of the evaluation, we'll call.

"Hey, douchebag." His voice rises. "Call my cousin, now."

I say nothing, remind myself that he's been popped with bullets. He's scared, anxious, maybe in shock. Or he's a thug, a power fiend, and now he's vulnerable and trying to maintain a measure of control. Or he distrusts authority, hates it, holds few reasons to believe the system cares about him. Maybe he is drunk. All these possibilities could be in play, or none of them.

His head rears off the stretcher and meets my eyes.

"Now, douchebag!"

I'm aware of the looks pinging between docs, nurses, and ER techs.

"Let us take care of you," I say, offering shared control, hoping he'll soften up and participate in his care.

He stares me down. He refuses IVs, bloods, imaging.

"What are we doing, douchebag? Are you calling my cousin or what?"

My stomach drops into a bottomless pit.

"What gives you the right to talk to us this way?" I finally say. "We're trying to help you." His eyes are cold and flat like steel rivets. I tear the blood pressure cuff from his right bicep. "Why am I fighting you? If you don't want to let us help you, you're free to go."

"What? You're kicking me out?"

"Good luck, sir."

"I'm calling my lawyer."

When he's gone, I neither swell with satisfaction nor sigh with relief. It's that word. Douchebag. I've been called plenty worse in my career. I'm aware that many health providers—in ERs, hospital wards, clinics, and offices—have been denigrated because of their gender, the color of their skin, their nationality or religion, their sexual preference, their age; and their abuse was worse than this instance by orders of magnitude. For reasons I can't explain, "douchebag," at that moment, crossed a line. I was left stone cold. And yet, I discovered that pushing him out the door left me feeling colder.

Kicking out a man from the ER during his initial evaluation for a gunshot wound is not only insensitive, unprofessional, and unethical; it reeks of medical-legal negligence. Fortunately for Mr. Blunt and me, the account I described is story truth, not happening truth. Tim O'Brien distinguishes "story" truth from "happening" truth in *The Things They Carried*. O'Brien writes: "By telling stories, you objectify your own experience. You separate it from yourself. You pin down certain truths. You make up others. You start sometimes with an incident that truly happened . . . and you carry it forward by inventing incidents that did not in fact occur but that nonetheless help to clarify and explain."

Years later, struggling to write an accurate account of this experience felt emotionally dishonest. I cared for a man with potentially critical wounds, a nasty attitude, and a fondness for the term "douchebag." Efforts by staff to soothe him were met with more insults. There were other injuries, and he told us exactly what we could do with our IVs, labs, imaging. He denied drinking, and his blood-alcohol level was more than two times higher than the legal limit. We sedated him, and by making him sleepy, we provided the diagnostic evaluation he needed and deserved. He was lucky; the gunshot wound was superficial. His head and shoulder were banged up, but nothing more. When daylight came around, he didn't say, "Thank you." But he stopped calling me douchebag. Sometimes, low-level ingratitude makes for a beautiful sunrise.

Emergency medicine was built on the pillars of "egalitarianism, social justice and compassion," caring for the marginalized and underserved in our healthcare system. The Emergency Medical Treatment and Active Labor Act (EMTALA) codified this ethos into statute. Every patient presenting to the ER can expect a screening exam for a medical emergency. Somehow, this obligation morphed over the years. The ER became a place where patients feel empowered to insult, threaten, and injure the very people on whom they're dependent for help. In turn, physicians, nurses, and other healthcare providers must not only absorb and accept their abuse, they are morally and legally bound to care for them. But how much tolerance is appropriate or psychologically healthy? What if a patient spits on us, or throws a urinal at a nurse, or takes the meal just served to them by an ER tech and chucks it on the floor?

In this situation, the desire to respect each patient with "common courtesy, sincerity, and willingness to help" competed against uglier feelings that questioned why we accept as normal the same behavior that gets people tossed from bars. While caring for Mr. Blunt, the happening truth was far less exciting than the agitation running beneath the surface of my care. Leaning on bedrock duties and virtues and patience didn't fill me with professional pride. What compelled me to write about this wasn't the word itself but the internal disturbance that never surfaced—the overwhelming urge to throw him out.

The evaluation and treatment of traumatic injuries in the ER, like Mr. Blunt's gunshot wounds, are protocol driven. This standardized process aims to uphold a level of quality and best practices to optimize the efficient care of trauma patients. The team shares a mutual understanding of what needs to happen at each step of the evaluation. Stomaching Mr. Blunt's personality and disrespect was part of that expectation.

There are different strategies for coping with insults from ER patients: (1) shake it off, (2) convince yourself you didn't hear what you did, and (3) pretend the loose slip of the tongue is a comment they'll later regret and apologize for. I've tried all of them. These good-faith reflexes give the patient the benefit of the doubt, and most of the time, such forgiveness is its reward. But sometimes, what we consider prudence is a cover for skirting what we should recognize and explore.

It might seem easier to lump people such as Mr. Blunt under familiar headings such as the "difficult patient." But I've found these shortcuts bypass the more difficult work of knowing individuals, their bonnets and bruises, and the conditions in that moment that are responsible for the behavior.

Medical expertise is born from repetition and accumulating experiences. But with routine experiences, we're inclined to shortcut our perceptions. As Viktor Shklovsky pointed out in his famous 1917 essay, we are less likely to see that which we frequently encounter. We see silhouettes, enough to identify and characterize. To truly recognize them again with all their particularity requires disorientation, or "making strange." Only by complicating our previous ways of knowing can we slow our perceptions and appreciate objects and experiences in a new way. Writing and the arts function as a medium for defamiliarization.

Writing properly about Mr. Blunt took years. Part of the difficulty wasn't only seeing inside Mr. Blunt's silhouette but getting past the blurred and softer impression of myself. By foregrounding the good care he received, I tended to give my raw and uncomfortable emotions a pass. Ultimately, I needed what Charles Baxter has called "misfit details," which resist our tendency for automatic looking. Running a scenario where I kicked out Mr. Blunt became the ultimate gesture of making strange. A dose of story truth lowered my psychic defenses. I finally gained access to previously suppressed emotions. Only by acknowledging these darker feelings at play in this charged moment could I take a measure of control over them.

By using the imagination as a moral testing ground, I built a bridge to future moments, echoed in words to a recent patient. "We will not tolerate your language or behavior, but we want to help you. We'll do our best to make you feel better. We're on your side."

Writing can't necessarily transform difficult patients into likable people. Still, the process served as a reminder of how hard it can be to understand another person and how the force of expectations and obligations may inadvertently prevent us from fully seeing ourselves. Beneath public faces are secret lives and bad days. I developed empathy for the character Mr. Blunt that I never felt for the actual person he represented. Mr. Blunt became more complex and relatable, allowing me to turn a heated encounter into an illuminating burn.

31
In Defense of Cheaper Stethoscopes

I was working alongside an emergency medicine colleague one evening when she surprised me with this confession: she'd been borrowing my stethoscope during ER shifts when I wasn't on duty. Her stethoscope had vanished months before, and she expressed no immediate plans to replace it. Our white coats shared the coat rack in a tiny room that smelled of whatever Tupperware-mystery was decomposing inside the minifridge. "The earpieces fit my ears just so," she said of my lower-end Littman, with its rubber missing from around the bell, then let out a gale-force sigh. "Your stethoscope has the spirit of an older physician."

Older physician? When did that happen? I hoped older implied a wiser physician, someone experienced enough not to waste money on a costly stethoscope.

This ER shift, she was using the magnificent acoustic instrument belonging to another ER physician in our group. "But it's a younger doc's stethoscope." A sly grin hid dismay. "It's not the same."

My colleague's missing stethoscope was as high-end as the one draped over her neck, though she was an older physician, too, and should have known better.

A dizzying assortment of objects have disappeared from ERs. Freshly poured coffee. Donuts sitting on napkins. White coats with the rightful owner's name stitched clearly over the breast pocket. Mobile phones. Purses. iPads and laptops. Waiting-room cardboard displays promoting services for sexually transmitted infections and substance use. Even heart monitors. Over the years I've lost my hair, a permanent state, along with my idealism, which graces me with frequent and quite pleasant visits. So many of my stethoscopes have gone AWOL that I've lost count. I've noted, however, that stethoscopes are subject to the same gravitational forces as sunglasses and pens. Expensive models float off into the darkest reaches of the galaxy. The modest, functional versions return home like boomerangs.

The ambient sounds that fill ERs—the monitors, the voices, the pain, the ringing phones, the pistons in my brain as I try to think—compete and coalesce into a blanket hum that complicates acoustics and negates the advantages of a premium stethoscope. When noise is everywhere, hearing isn't the problem, but *not* hearing: sorting through the sounds and voices, knowing what to tune out and tune in, and hoping you're making the right choices.

When René Laennec, the French physician and inventor of the stethoscope, rolled a sheath of papers to conduct the chest sounds of a young woman on rounds in 1816, he ushered in a vibrant era of modern medicine. Derived from the Greek *stethos* for "chest" and *skopos* for "observer," the stethoscope has symbolized my chosen career more than any other instrument. The stethoscope I received on entering medical school embodied all the knowledge and skills I was responsible to master. It represented the gravity and immensity of my future life's work, more so than the white coat, which always felt like a starchy straitjacket, a persona that never fit me properly.

The stethoscope is more than a piece of medical equipment. It provides an opportunity for personal expression. Pediatricians hang furry creatures from the tubing like it's a tree limb in paradise. Young physicians sport delicious colors such as raspberry, peach, and orange. Physicians who served with the Indian Health Service often adorn their tubing in intricate, Native American handiwork, like tight sweaters on handbag dogs. Internists and cardiologists bear the stethoscope with a quiet swagger, as if it's Indiana Jones's whip, a tool capable of rooting out the wiliest heart murmur, disarming the most combative surgeon, and pulling them out from a pit of poisonous snakes. The orthopedists, meanwhile, stride like proud nudists, not knowing when the last time they wore a stethoscope or where it was hidden should they ever need it.

For those of us who use a stethoscope as part of our daily work, it becomes a body part. That my colleague found comfort placing my earpieces inside her ears made me uneasy. It's hard to explain. Our relationship with certain objects can become personal, and they don't share well with others for reasons that aren't always logical. Baseball hat? Sure. Baseball mitt? Umm. A five iron? Go ahead. A putter? Over my dead body. Shirt? I guess. Underwear? Yuck. I'm fascinated by the transgressions I accept as normal. For example,

I tolerate the odors, secretions, and decay of sick and unfortunate bodies in my work, and yet I get the creeps each time I squeeze my feet into rented bowling shoes.

So much of being a physician involves sharing experiences, both personal and clinical, that are disorienting: mistakes in judgment or behavior; opportunities lost through doubt or fear or fatigue; even successes that shocked us. The expanse of medicine is daunting and complicated. We must, by necessity, learn from the experiences of others. Medical school and residency for me involved being on call every third or every fourth night, but many of my teachers boasted of working every other night at the hospital. They'd ask, "Do you know the worst part of being on call every other night?" The answer was always: "You miss half the interesting cases."

My stethoscope had acquired talismanic properties, time-earned luck, along with a memory of the thousands of patients we'd listened to together. During critical moments when uncertainty or panic pushed into my head, my trusted stethoscope helped focus my attention. Slow down and close your eyes, it advised me. We've been here before. Listen to what the body is telling you, and what it's not.

With time, the stethoscope becomes your child, and a loving, responsible parent doesn't share his child with anyone else. But my colleague had my blessing to continue plundering the pocket of my white coat. She's a wonderful parent. She and her partner have all boys, and one has autism spectrum disorder. She has the patience, the resolve, the tested love that makes me strive to be a better person. Wouldn't my stethoscope benefit from working with someone more understanding and patient, who engaged the most challenging patients without judgment or an edge to her voice?

In turn, when my stethoscope sat around my neck, I could channel my colleague's nuclear-powered empathy. The stethoscope we shared didn't make me a better doctor; it allowed me to tap into that place in me where a more emotionally evolved doctor could be found.

Regardless of how old, wise, or kind you are, there is always room to do it better the next time. To that end, you must listen to your own heart before you can listen to others. It starts with relinquishing ego. Becoming an older physician requires being humbled again and again. The body doesn't read the textbooks, and it's safe to assume patients haven't read the script you want them to follow. There's only one true way to become an excellent doctor, and that's to take care of patients, an endless train of them. And when each situation feels new and particular, unsettling and surprising, you must be open to being startled.

Teachable moments and pricks of insight often strike without warning, usually outside the knowledge delivery systems such as lecture halls and ward rounds. Nurses and ward clerks, social workers and translators, security guards and housekeepers have all been my teachers. They have offered winking approvals and cast a hot spotlight on behaviors, attitudes, and actions that "weren't me."

Patients have been my greatest teachers: this is how you die with grace; this is how you survive on the streets; this is how you don't talk to me; this is how you earn my trust.

When I first entered medical school, awestruck by the stethoscope, I never imagined the most influential teacher in my medical career would come in the form of the late Walter James Miller, an New York University professor, author, and poet. He was not a physician. His mentorship, and later friendship, began during my year away from medical school to write. He knew that to write well, you must first write poorly. But you must write. He rarely took a sharp knife to my prose though it deserved a samurai. Years later, I accused him of being too kind to my early work. He said I wasn't ready for that type and depth of criticism. First, I needed encouragement, room to find my voice, and permission to stay true to what he knew was so important to me. He shepherded the conditions so I could discover what I needed to learn. Only now, thirty years later, do I recognize mentoring so deftly wrought I didn't know it was going on. I've "borrowed" more from his mentoring style than from any other physician/educator.

I'm now an older physician and still a work in progress, thirsty for ways to become a better version of myself.

What does this have to do with my beat-up stethoscope?

Despite its many functions as instrument, adornment, and friend, my cheaper stethoscope is limited as a unidirectional conductor of the body's sounds. It captures narrative fragments, tiny statements. What matters is how we translate these sounds, intellectually and emotionally, into meaningful action. Listening through and around the earpieces of my cheaper stethoscope—an idea that winks at Laennec's original definition of the stethoscope as a chest observer—might offer the best way to reconcile sound, silence, and suggestion into a coherent story.

There are dangers to becoming a high-end stethoscope. The writer/critic Anatole Broyard said it best: "There is a paradox here at the heart of medicine, because a doctor, like a writer, must have a voice of his own, something that conveys the timbre, the rhythm, the diction, and the music of his humanity that compensates us for all the speechless machines."

Eric Topol, a world-renowned cardiologist and thinker on the transformational role of technology in medicine, called the stethoscope nothing more than a pair of "rubber tubes." The next-generation stethoscope is an ultrasound machine that transmits images to a screen, not sounds to our ears. Instead of detecting a heart murmur and connecting it to the anatomical abnormality it signifies, we can visualize the anatomy directly. But the body isn't replicated like a photograph; it's represented on the screen as acoustic signals in a spectrum of white, black, and grays. The details are identified through skilled interpretation of shadows.

I frequently wonder whether the death knell for the stethoscope isn't too far off, and the next time my stethoscope vanishes, should I bother replacing it?

This isn't a theoretical question. The COVID-19 pandemic has changed how we use the stethoscope. We've altered acceptable practices to minimize the risk of infecting ourselves or transmitting the SARS-CoV-2 virus to others. Most stethoscopes aren't six feet long. If we need to, we use disposable versions that we assemble and keep in the room. I suspect Laennec's rolled sheath of papers worked better as a transmitter of sound. But when a patient is working hard to breathe, it feels awkward and irresponsible not to place a stethoscope to their chest. For all the diagnostic utility of ultrasound, especially during the pandemic, it lacks the iconic force of the stethoscope. The ultrasound can pick up fluid around the heart and lungs, detect how strong the heart is pumping, but the stethoscope speaks to patients— I'm right here.

The practice of medicine is nuanced and oblique. It needs personalities willing to take fully authentic breaths. Better technology won't necessarily replace what humans need most from each other: the promise of connection. I might not be perfect, but I'll be present. After all these years, I'm still working on finding my voice in medicine. Patients continue to surprise me, and as a consequence, I continue to surprise myself. I've become more comfortable with that, as I was with sharing a stethoscope with a colleague I respect so much. She eventually moved on to another job that rewarded her remarkable clinical and teaching skills, and I moved on as well. My stethoscope vanished. I'd like to imagine a younger physician using it, channeling the experience of two older physicians while acquiring and accumulating their own, but I'm doubtful. It was only a fair conductor of pure sounds. But if you knew what to listen for, there was no better guide.

32
The Appendix: Ancient Organ for the Modern Age

The appendix is a body part with an image problem. Derived from the Latin word for "hanging on," the term can mean a bodily outgrowth or a supplementary material attached at the end of a document. The anatomical appendix is a tubular sac tagged on to the lower end of the colon. The point being, it's extra—tolerated, but never celebrated.

Poets rarely, if ever, invoke the appendix with the passion reserved for the heart. The brain and the mind can rest for eternity on the lofty "I think, therefore I am." The eyes have been hailed as the doorway to love and the windows to the soul. The appendix, however, is a humble organ of lymphoid tissue.

The lymphatic system works as the body's infection-fighting network, but remove the appendix and the immune system still functions quite well. Taking out the spleen, also composed of lymphoid tissue, creates a susceptibility to certain bacterial infections. The spleen's absence can change people's identity. Should they become sick, doctors consider them immunocompromised.

The appendix, like many body parts, earns our attention only when it misbehaves. Appendicitis, an angry state when the walls swell and turn inflamed, can produce intolerable abdominal pain. After this harsh introduction, the surgeon typically comes in and calmly assures us we'll feel better once it's gone.

Convincing someone, anyone, to lament its loss is a tall order. The appendix is a vestigial organ whose moment of glory belongs in the long-forgotten evolutionary past and must now fight for relevance and self-worth. But what if there's more to this tubular ribbon than anatomy and physiology? Almost thirty years into a life in emergency medicine, I've been asking myself, "What if I am an appendix, facing similar challenges and perhaps, similar fates?"

There is an old medical aphorism: "Heal sometimes, treat often, comfort always." For much of my career, I could be downright arrogant in my belief that nothing could rival the moral force of caring for patients.

Today, this nugget has become: "Contribute to the profit margin always, document to maximize billing, comfort if you have the time." My value as a doctor in the modern healthcare enterprise is a product of multiple factors, including the number of patients I see, how quickly I see them after they hit the door, and how much revenue I generate. My worth is highlighted on spreadsheets and bar graphs and pie charts.

Left out are skills more difficult to measure, such as how well I listen, my ability to connect, whether I turn away or acknowledge my patient's struggles even if I can't alleviate them.

I'm monitored by yardsticks that look at health quality in particular and often contradictory ways. For example, I receive a slap on the wrist if I don't start antibiotics early in patients whose vital signs point to possible sepsis. But if another explanation arises to explain those findings, and the patient doesn't have a blood infection, I'm faulted for prescribing antibiotics unnecessarily and contributing to the antibiotic resistance problem.

The disconnect between what patients value and what the system expects of me leaves me feeling appendiceal. A misplaced and outdated cog in a healthcare system that treats patients as commodities while it counts on physicians to remain moral creatures, to adhere to the ancient precept, "The patient always comes first."

In the modern age, the dogged persistence of the appendix is a source of inspiration. Hundreds of thousands of years into the human experiment, the appendix is still with us. Along the way, the body has ruthlessly shed much of what was considered unnecessary. Tail? Gone. Gills? Extraneous to life on land and a challenge to garments with sleeves.

Researchers claim the appendix has evolved over thirty different times across multiple species. Recent evidence suggests it serves a previously unknown function as a vital reservoir for gut bacteria. This discovery might earn the appendix its "Rocky" moment. Even so, I believe its real value isn't medical but metaphorical.

The appendix is a stubborn reminder that we must remain defiant when we feel irrelevant, ignored, and valued only as lines on a spreadsheet. During every clinical encounter, an act of rebellion is to ask yourself, "How do I do what's best for this patient?"

In the not-too-distant future, the time will come for me to leave emergency medicine. After I'm gone, after goodbye drinks and the sharing of old stories, the system will grind on just fine without me. Whenever I think of that, I can't blame the appendix for making a little noise before getting cut from the body.

Maybe the gallbladder is a better anatomical comparison to my present state. It's a globular sac that spits out bile and breaks down fatty foods. The body functions well without it, too, though it's not necessarily forgotten. Overindulging in that cheesesteak will quickly remind you of its absence.

We all hit against moments when we question how we derive meaning in our lives. To this end, the vestigial appendix excels as a crafty provocateur. It demonstrates how there's nobility in hanging on, sticking around, and even being a pest. It challenges us to continually examine what we value in ourselves and others and why. The appendix is worthy of a poem or two.

33
Judging Patients

Mrs. Gomes, my umpteenth patient of the day, is an older woman—only slightly older than myself—who came to the emergency department with a cough, an upset stomach, and diarrhea.

Compared to the train of patients with known and suspected COVID-19, she belongs in the tired but otherwise well-appearing camp. There are no worrisome findings on her physical exam: a borderline fever, a reassuring oxygen saturation level, and a chest X-ray without the worrisome white puffs and fingerlike haziness common in the lower lungs of patients with COVID-19 pneumonia. After receiving a few liters of intravenous fluid, Mrs. Gomes is eager to go home.

I move my N95 mask off the pressure sore on my nose and tell her that she'll learn the results of her COVID-19 test in a day or two. In the meantime, she should keep her face covered and self-quarantine. She scrunches her brows, then plays with her face mask. "But I'm supposed to visit my daughter," she tells me.

Her daughter, I learn, lives a plane flight away.

Though we are waiting on the test results, I suspect from her symptoms, and the accompanying fatigue, that she'll test positive for COVID-19.

"You shouldn't be traveling for the holidays," I say, raising my voice. "You likely have COVID-19."

"What?" she yelps.

Over the N95 mask I wear a surgical mask, and a face shield in front of them. These necessary layers of protection echo my normal speaking voice back to me. What's loud to my ears is heard as incomprehensible mumbling to patients. Turning up the volume has become part of everyday communication, which doesn't feel right in situations like this one when I actually feel like screaming.

How could she travel for the holidays during a pandemic in which the daily national death toll makes each day feel like 9/11? The constant influx of very sick patients stresses hospital capacity across the United States and imposes unbearable burdens on health care workers.

Gripped by this frightening reality, I feel my tone leaking with judgment. Mrs. Gomes seems to be a kind person. I regret the edge to my voice and brace for a well-deserved sharp retort from her.

During this second surge, I no longer feel as noble and inspired as I did last spring. When I'm tired, there's a tendency to be critical of patients such as Mrs. Gomes, whose actions feed this unprecedented crisis. Admitting this leaves me embarrassed, especially when I notice the severity and purity of her disappointment, like that of a child whose ice cream has fallen to the sidewalk.

"I'll wear a facemask when I'm there," she says. "Promise."

Behind layers of protection, my interactions with patients feel dampened of nuance. Despite all that's covered, there's a wealth of texture revealed in the window above the cheeks. From behind Mrs. Gomes's window, I read an expression of sadness and longing.

I explain to Mrs. Gomes how, if she has COVID-19, she could infect people in the airport, on the plane, and in her daughter's house. She doesn't argue with me. I'm impressed by the precautions she's taken to date. She lives alone and goes out in public only to shop for food and take the occasional walk. She clearly recognizes the risk of infecting others, and the dangers of virus transmission in indoor spaces with proximity to others. But she recently attended a birthday party with relatives, some of whom weren't wearing masks. Somehow, family is different from the public. Her contact with family counted as a different type of engagement, as if shared DNA or familial connections provided a containment against the virus.

"I won't be leaving my daughter's house," she says. "I'll be spending a few days at home with my daughter and grandchildren."

I rub my nose through my masks. A low-level headache taps between my eyes. I can barely take the weight of the thin wire-rimmed eyeglasses perched on my face.

"But if you have COVID, you're the one they should be distanced from. You're putting your daughter and her family at risk."

There's so much attention on the extremes of responses in this pandemic. Defiant people refuse to wear facial coverings or social distance based on political affiliations, conspiracy theories, personal beliefs, and misinformation. Less often do we talk about what seems to be irresponsible behavior that doesn't fit into neat categories.

In my many conversations with patients in the ER, it is this other group, which defies familiar classification, that is more common.

Social distancing is a problem in this pandemic. But so is the distance between knowledge and our lives, our assessment of risk and our needs. Mrs. Gomes is worried about becoming infected with COVID-19, yet the odds of her transmitting it to others didn't match her need to see her family.

Like many of my patients, Mrs. Gomes isn't being unreasonable or irrational. They're realists, struggling to balance the reality in which they're living. I've cared for several patients with COVID-19, or who have signs and symptoms of the disease and awaiting test results, who are more terrified of missed paychecks than a virus. They had mouths to feed, rent to pay, and hope for something extra for holiday gifts. I argue with them the way I make my case with Mrs. Gomes.

I'm learning that it's laziness to judge their behavior, to assume they're selfish or unwilling to sacrifice personal comforts for the greater good. Part of me wants to tell Mrs. Gomes that it's dangerous for her to get on that plane. But she already knows that. Educating her about COVID-19 requires more than knowledge about the virus and protective measures against it. Scientific evidence isn't enough.

For all its lethality and social destruction, the coronavirus isn't the only big problem in many of my patient's lives. It's one of many. Patients make decisions for reasons that aren't immediately clear to outsiders. This is not to say there aren't those who congregate irresponsibly in large groups at parties, clubs, beaches, and seats of government power. They have a heavy hand in the record numbers of cases and the rising death toll.

Mrs. Gomes hadn't seen her daughter and her family in many, many months. It was love—not selfishness—that blinded her ability to recognize that she had become a threat to their health and the health of others. Her love for her family was worth dying over. But unsuspecting others may suffer because of that love.

Because it takes extra effort and time, both in short supply during the pandemic, it's easier for health care providers like me to lump the perceived resisters into a large category of misbehavior rather than weighing the risks of getting or spreading COVID-19 on balance with the other risks.

Trying to understand people's motivations and to withhold judgment along the way isn't easy, so we best get to work. When COVID-19 is finally behind us—and I pray that time comes soon—parsing out the questions of "why" with sensitivity and clarity will become necessary for building a healthier society.

34
A Knock on the Door

"I'm sorry," I say, pulling up a chair. I offer my hand. "I can't tell you how sorry I am."

Mrs. H sits exhausted and empty on a chair next to the stretcher, her winter coat buttoned to the neck, clutching her handbag. She tugs at the wool cap sitting over her ears. She stares at my hand and nods.

Her son, a young boy, has just died in the children's hospital next door. She screamed and fought off everyone who tried to console her when she heard the news. She's my patient because the family felt she needed something to help calm her.

I have tissues and time.

My baby my baby my baby my baby my baby . . .

Her cousin motions that we should step into the corridor. She's dressed like Mrs. H, bundled up against the chill. She fills in the details.

A knock on the front door. Then gunshots. The boy wasn't the intended target, the cousin said. Gang-related, the police suspect. A mistake. The wrong house, the wrong victim. An alarming statement that implies there's such a thing as the right house and the right victim.

I sense Mrs. H heard what her cousin has said. When we return, she says, "Why did I open the door?"

There are over a quarter-million words in the English language and yet I can't find a single word for Mrs. H that feels appropriate. After years of practice, rare are the moments when any expression of solace rings hollow.

"Why wouldn't you open the door," I wanted to say. There are many reasons why Mrs. H wouldn't open the door, except isn't that what neighbors do?

"Why?" Mrs. H. argues silently to herself.

My baby my baby my baby my baby my baby . . .

These words dance lightly on her lips. She chokes up, fights back tears, and retreats into an impenetrable silence. My presence is all I can offer even when I know it's not enough.

My baby my baby my baby my baby my baby . . .

These words hang in the air, pull me into a cavernous space that's connected to every parent's nightmare.

I ask Mrs. H if I can get her anything. Maybe a glass of water? She's not thirsty. We bring water anyway, not because she'll feel better but because it's an action, a distraction. It makes us feel less inadequate, our powerlessness less terrifying.

My baby my baby my baby my baby my baby . . .

Mrs. H has another child, a younger son. She had protected them both well enough until this evening, after supper, when there was a knock on the door.

35
Paper Scrubs

I spent my first on-call overnights with the surgery team placing IVs, drawing blood, chasing lab results, and fetching White Castle sliders, so I jumped when Dr. Allen told me to haul my ass down to the ER. Staff was spilling into the trauma room, blocking my view of the patient. A horrific car crash. The patient had hurled through the driver's side windshield. And yet, the surgery residents and nurses worked slowly, wearing blunted expressions I didn't expect. Sleeplessness, perhaps, but there was a stricken quality, too. I was desperate for a better angle, a closer look. Then Dr. Allen barked my name. "Where's the student?"

That's what Dr. Allen, the chief surgical resident, called all third-year medical students in the first weeks of our surgery clerkship in the thick of July, in the late 1980s.

In this tired city hospital in Queens, New York, the air conditioning was lazy, the wards steamy, and the scrubs made of paper. Such scrubs were the fate of students who didn't own more comfortable and concealing fabrics. If you sweat, it showed. The sound of my name turned me into a faucet of anxiety.

"Put a gown on him," said Dr. Allen.

A hand pressed a gown into my chest. My sweaty arms got stuck in the sleeves.

"What's the holdup?"

Latex gloves. The booties didn't slide easily over my suede buck shoes.

"Next to me," Dr. Allen insisted.

The crowd stepped aside. My legs didn't want to move.

Earlier that week, while Dr. Allen was operating and I was retracting, he'd swung the overhead lamp and clocked me in the head. I was tall, and he wasn't. Dr. Allen never looked up from the surgical field. Afterward, I nerved up and mentioned what had happened. He stared off. Perhaps he'd heard me, and didn't care. Maybe he was deep in thought, and it didn't register. Those first few weeks were a never-ending collision with everything I didn't know.

"Closer," Dr. Allen said.

Slow your breathing, I told myself, taking note of the overhead lamp and then looking down. I couldn't reach the patient without stepping on the blood-streaked tiles. My feet felt wet and sticky without being wet and sticky. Then my eyes landed on the patient's chest, or what was left of it. Carved open, ribs spread like a clamshell. And the heart. Dr. Allen was squeezing this man's heart. My lungs hurt.

"Ever do direct cardiac massage before?" Dr. Allen said, in a manner that assumed the answer, of course, was no. He took my gloved hands, placed them above and behind the heart. He adjusted my fingers. "Now count," he said. "One and two and . . ."

Was I squeezing the human heart? I had held the heart in the anatomy lab, dissected it, committed to memory the chambers, valves, and vessels. But this was the first time I felt the heart, recognized it as a muscle. And it was warm. Could he be alive? I was sweating, wet with awe and terror. But inside the terror, I lost track of time and found focus and a super-saturated clarity never experienced before. I raised my eyes for Dr. Allen's approval. Hand position? Rate of my compressions? But he was gone. Everyone was gone.

Panic took over. "Where's Dr. Allen?"

"Talking with the family," said the lone nurse, preoccupied with charting.

Before I could ask another question, Dr. Allen burst into the trauma room. "Stop," he said. "Close him up."

"What?"

"Suture the chest. Big bites. Nothing fancy."

"Wait!"

"See you upstairs when you're done."

My excitement melted. I wasn't saving a life; I was resuscitating a dead man.

By directing my attention entirely to the act of cardiac message, I missed the intestines dangling out of the patient's chest and the purpose of what seemed to be a futile act.

I was hot with embarrassment. A massive force must rupture the diaphragm for the bowel to enter the chest. The nurse clunked down the suture tray laid out with thick nylon sutures attached to needles the size of spears. "Here you go."

"Sure," I said, feigning confidence.

I hadn't sutured much. But I was disturbed less by what I couldn't do than by what I wasn't feeling. Where was the shock each time the slippery intestines sprung to the floor as I gathered it into the chest? What about disgust? Frustration mounted, but it quickly registered as an everyday frustration. As if I wasn't doing something gruesome but something routine, like tugging on a knotted garden hose.

Once I set out suturing, the chest came together, albeit awkwardly. Forcing the needle into the ribcage took force. Squaring the knots become a fumbling exercise. Once finished, I squared the crooked and uneven sutures with intense relief, even joy. I'd accomplished a task I couldn't have imagined when the night began. But beneath the ecstasy was the fear I'd lost something, too.

I heard cries from outside the closed trauma room doors and signaled to the nurse. She nodded toward the body. "His family."

This patient, whose face was so bruised and deformed, had been a person hours before. A person with a family.

"You first hearing that?" she whispered.

I had heard these cries but I couldn't locate them. They belonged to the ambient noises of a busy ER at nighttime, a human jungle where suffering appeared everywhere and thus registered as nowhere, making it easier to ignore.

I washed up and slumped out of the trauma room. The sunrise hurt my eyes as I passed the glass windows by the ambulance bay and plodded down the corridor, my back stiff from leaning over for such a long period.

"Doctor?" I heard behind me. I waited for a reply from around an unseen corner or stairwell. It was an urgent female voice, and it followed me as I walked toward the elevator. "Doctor?"

I couldn't be the "doctor" she was after. I stopped and turned. The woman appeared to be about my age, except the tears had washed away any traces of youth. The patient's wife introduced herself, then she swallowed, steadied herself, and hit me with two words I never expected to hear. "Thank you." She was grateful for everything I'd done for her husband.

I was speechless. My first impulse was to set things straight, tell her I'm not a doctor, urge her to look at my paper scrubs, soaked through and barely holding together. But what if she asked what I'd been doing all this time. Could I say I was a medical student learning on her husband? That evening's adrenaline rush washed away. My body ached, now. A headache fogged my eyes.

I thought for a second, then a few seconds more. "I'm sorry for your loss," I finally said, a safe and disappointing reply, mechanical words of comfort when you don't know what to say. A child in pajamas could have done better. It didn't require expertise, only a warm, beating heart. But I was an insecure medical student in paper scrubs, too focused on not saying the wrong words instead of reaching out like a fellow human.

When I found my way onto the wards to prepare for morning rounds, Dr. Allen said I had learned skills to care for the next trauma patient. Maybe so, but I couldn't stop thinking about the patient's wife. What was she doing when I had been called to the trauma room? The night was winding down. If they had children, she probably had just put them to bed and maybe was stealing quiet time reading or catching up on work or enjoying a mug of tea or glass of wine. Or maybe she had been chatting on the phone with friends or relatives. I'll never know, and decades later, my imagination can't stop spinning scenarios. More comfortable fabrics can't protect me from the one truth I know for sure, and that haunts me to this day. I hadn't served her husband; her husband served me. I'll never forget that night. It was the first time I felt like a doctor, and that memory isn't possible unless a family also remembers it, only as a nightmare when their lives, hopes, and dreams are changed forever.

36
The Ashtray

It was morning rounds, the first day of the first month of my internship, the very beginning of my emergency medicine training, over thirty years ago. The ink on my medical diploma was barely dry, and I was part of the medical intensive care unit (MICU) team, responsible for some of the sickest patients in the medical center. I'd just picked up Mrs. Andrews's care, who was on life support for a lung infection that spread to her bloodstream. A ventilator had kept her alive for weeks while a changing cocktail of antibiotics dripped into her veins. I could see my nerves in the shaky handwriting as I squeezed the details of her rocky course onto an index card.

I sighed relief when I learned Mrs. Andrews's infection was improving, but that comfort quickly evaporated. Emphysema from years of cigarettes had damaged her lungs, and the MICU team couldn't get her off the ventilator. Her family—a husband and several adult children—weren't too pleased that we hadn't pulled the breathing tube. Hadn't we said she was better?

They made their displeasure and confusion known to me soon after I introduced myself as the new intern. I stumbled through an explanation. The chest wall and the diaphragm expand when we inhale, creating a negative pressure that enables the lungs to breathe in. When the ventilator took over for Mrs. Andrews, the chest and diaphragm muscles grew weak from lack of use. Yes, the infection in her lungs had improved, but tests showed her chest muscles weren't strong enough. She wasn't ready to breathe on her own. She would die. They nodded, then said: "But she wants the tube out."

A few days passed. Each morning I'd visit Mrs. Andrews and she'd motion with her hands how she wanted me to please remove the tube. Then the family would arrive and ask to speak to me. "What about the breathing tube?"

Whenever we gave her a trial to see if she was strong enough to fly on her own, it was clear she wasn't strong enough yet. Mrs. Andrews and her family understood what we said, even accepted it, while at the same time pressing us with polite disagreement. They sensed my insecurities, I feared. They smelled "new doctor." My ID badge was unscratched, my white coat stiff and blindingly white. But I was fortified by the accumulated experiences of my senior medical resident and the supervising ICU director, who to this day stand as some of the brightest physicians I've worked with.

To my surprise, the family didn't debate the facts. And they spoke with an appreciation for the treatment team's breadth of expertise. In their eyes, the issue wasn't our medical expertise, but everything we didn't know about Mrs. Andrews.

Later that week, I arrived on the MICU in the morning to discover Mrs. Andrews sitting up in bed, the breathing tube out, sucking on ice chips.

She waved and flashed me a devilish smile. But the nurse looked worried. "Overnight, she yanked the tube out. Enough's enough."

My gut flipped, then knotted.

"Mrs. Andrews," I said, "you're not ready."

She flew her open palms up as if to say, "Look at me."

"But you'll tire out. And when that happens . . . You can die without the tube."

Mrs. Andrews could barely speak, her voice hoarse from weeks of a breathing tube wedged between her vocal cords, but she made herself clear. 'No more tubes.'

I wanted to scream, to puke, to cry. How could Mrs. Andrews be so irresponsible? But when the family came into the MICU, they were elated. I asked them to talk to her. She's made her wishes painfully clear, they said.

There was little I could do but wait. Nervously wait. I checked on her between visits with my other patients that morning, reduced to the role of a scared cheerleader. I recited an incantation to myself. Don't die. Don't die. Please, don't die.

I couldn't shake the feeling that I'd messed up and hadn't explained the situation well enough and Mrs. Andrews could die as a result. The nurse caring for her insisted it wasn't my fault. It was Mrs. Andrews's will.

Mrs. Andrews fed me a healthy diet of "I told you so" looks throughout that long day, and soon I began questioning my caution. Maybe it was my discomfort with risk, which exerted its own negative pressure and influenced how I'd framed the discussions with them. Regardless, by nightfall, the senior physicians moved her out of the MICU. "She gambled and won," they said. "Good for her."

A month later, one of Mrs. Andrews's daughters tracked me down in the ER, my next rotation, and pushed into my hands a small, gift-wrapped box.

Inside was a clear plastic ashtray encased around a needlepoint of the famous symbol of healing, the Greek staff of Hermes, a caduceus, entwined with two serpents. "My mom made it," she said. "It's a gift."

I was speechless. I couldn't imagine the time and effort required to make this. I explained that I couldn't accept this gift from a patient. It was unethical. Thank you, I said, and tried to push it back.

"You must take it."

"But . . ."

"My mom can be stubborn. You know that."

That evening, my smile was so wide it hurt as I placed the ashtray on my desk in my rented apartment. Mrs. Andrews and I both survived our month in the ICU. However, she didn't get better because of me but in spite of me. That thought chased me throughout my internship year.

As I moved forward with my career, I began to see this gift more literally—Mrs. Andrews gave me an ashtray! A patient with bad chronic lung disease due to a lifetime of cigarettes gave her doctor an ashtray. She still smoked, her daughter said, with a stern frown. But I bit my tongue because the hard-headedness that contributed to her critical illness probably played a hand in her recovery, too.

My relationship with this ashtray has spanned many decades—it's kept me company on every office desk I've ever had—and it continues to reveal itself as I've moved through my career. Recently, I reconsidered the "MD!!" stitched beneath my name. Why exclamation points, and why two? Does it applaud the achievement of becoming a doctor, or does the double strike undermine itself, make the argument that there's so much a doctor doesn't know? What she desperately needed from me—someone with the courage to understand her—isn't mastered in medical school, but in life. The enduring power of the ashtray rests in its mystery, a reminder that meaning unfolds slowly and emerges when you're ready to embrace it.

37
The Patient Who Wanted Nothing

My initial inquiries, "What can I do for you?" and "What brings you to the ER?" earn a sigh from Sadie M. Her leather tongue licks at raw lips that are painfully dry. She turns away, strings of graying hair loose against the stretcher pillow. Her look spells more than inexpressible fatigue. I suspect she's so far into her illness, she welcomes death more than she needs me. And should her condition earn her any privileges, it's the choice not to participate in doctor–patient theater.

From a seat in the corner, Sadie M's sister speaks as if nervous about trespassing into this fortress of silence. "It hurts to eat. Or drink," the sister says. When I suggest IV fluids might help her feel better, Sadie M holds out her thin arms, bruised from countless IVs, chemotherapy infusions and blood draws. Running IV fluid will require a deeper vein. Then she catches me spying her neck. "Don't even think about it," she whispers.

A few weeks earlier, Sadie M. left the hospital against the doctor's advice. She dropped out of hospice. Dropped out. What does that mean? Now, at this late hour, she comes to the ER. The complaint: "Not feeling right."

"Can you be more specific?"

I desperately want to help her. She's not even fifty, but years are a poor metric for what her body has endured. The whites of her eyes are jaundiced. So is the look she gives me.

"Help? I don't need your help."

Through raised eyebrows and pursed lips, her sister begs me to do something, please! Her medical record chronicles the details of her battle with metastatic breast cancer. And yet, despite everything I know about Sadie M's case, the endless catalog of tests and treatments, I have no grip on her story.

A medical case shouldn't be confused with a patient's story. A case presents a problem, and our job is to find the solution: What happened? What hurts? What makes it better or worse? But a story is about a person who struggles. Stories ask "Why?" They're concerned with the motivating forces driving a person's actions and behavior. Thinking meaningfully about a patient's story requires the imagination to venture beyond what "is" and into the realm of what "could" and "might" be.

Late evening, when the ER is exploding, isn't the ideal time for such deep contemplation. Sadie M is dying. She cut short her last hospital stay, left against the advice of her doctors, and now she's back and won't explain why. I should be satisfied with what little she offers, and do what I can. But there has to be a "why" for her visit. I can't ignore the mystery in her story.

I offer her juice and ginger ale and then remember that the day's supply of ginger ale is typically all gone at this hour. "How about cranberry or apple juice?"

"Apple juice? I'm not here for no juice."

We both dredge up sighs. Finally, I recruit her sister for help. "Sadie?" she says. "Talk to the doctor."

I ask about her day, up to the moment she decided to come to the ER. This information she is eager to share. That evening, she called her doctor's group and left several messages. Each call drained her of what little energy she had left. First, the instructions to call 911 if you have an emergency, then the heartless artificial voices followed by the gauntlet of options before finally reaching the prompt to leave a message and someone will call back. "Nobody called back," she says, seething.

I sense from her sister's eye-roll the scene wasn't pretty.

"When my doctor first told me about the lump, he said we were going through this together. When it got real bad and I said enough chemo, no more, where's he at? I don't see him."

Raspy outrage, but she's talking now. She tells me an unspooling of disappointments, troubles with her kids and grandkids. I let her go on, hoping the reason she's here would spill out. She mumbles something about wanting to punch the hospice nurse when there's a lurching stop. A trail of breathlessness cuts through the silence. She's tired. We can't underestimate the demands of speech.

Notes from doctors, social workers, and mental health counselors allude to her being difficult, describe meetings with Sadie M that ended abruptly. But Sadie M wasn't always fighting. Notes from earlier in her illness describe her as "pleasant." What happened?

Difficult patients are often people with stories where much is left out, and somewhere in the unspoken are their deepest fears. To access that portal, you must be on the look-out for it. But you're never completely sure that space exists and, if an invitation comes, what form it will take.

I fix my gaze on Sadie M. She turns to meet me, then quickly pulls away. She looks like a felled sparrow. But her sister boasts how she was once a bulldog. She raised her kids as a single mom. She is a fighter, someone who punched first and asked questions later, her sister says. This unexpected phrase makes me chuckle. Sadie M cuts me a look.

"You want me to show you?"

"Stop that," her sister whispers. I detect a hint of apology in her tone. Whether it's for my benefit or Sadie M's, I can't decide.

Sadie M brushes her sister away. She's not interested in medications to ease her pain or calm her nausea. When a patient appears to close off access to what I suspect is a key part of their story, I try a seemingly unrelated question. I ask Sadie M my "magic wand" question: "If I had a magic wand with the power to fix any problem for you, what might that be?"

I expect her to say kick cancer. Instead, she says. "I don't want to die like this."

I lower my head.

"Can I give you a hand in this fight?"

"What? You don't think I got this?"

This is the line I didn't know I was looking for. Behind her question was an assertion. What if her problem isn't her cancer or her dehydration? In fact, there's a school of thought that dehydration is a natural part of the dying process. What if what she needs from me is more fundamental, and it's been in plain sight the entire time? She wants recognition as the protagonist of her story.

We focus so much on diagnosis and treatment, on doing things to and for patients, but our best efforts can amount to misdirected diligence. Sometimes, the treatment is to safely return patients, not their diseases, to the center of their stories.

When I ask Sadie M why she dropped out of hospice, she describes how she hated the way doctors talked about comfort care. Being made comfortable implied passivity, not relief from physical and emotional distress. She lived her life fighting, and she wanted to die the same way.

"This is a hard fight for anyone."

Her jaw stiffens. I can't tell whether she is about to cry or throw a left hook.

"Maybe you can give her something for nausea. She needs to eat. To keep her strength."

Sadie M nods at her sister's request.

She lets me give her a dose of morphine, too, but she insists I send her home immediately after.

The next day, Sadie M died. Had she known the end was near? I suspect she had. I never discovered the reason behind her emergency visit. She never told me. My guess is she wanted to make one last stand. She might have lost a battle with cancer, but that wasn't going to stop her from picking another fight.

38
Can We Write a Better Story for Ourselves?

The Doctor, an iconic painting by Sir Luke Fildes, depicts a grave, regally bearded doctor in a tailored suit sitting beside a sick boy laid out across two chairs. In the background of the nineteenth-century English cottage stand the boy's parents, anxiously watching. But the viewer's attention is drawn to the devoted doctor, chin in hand, and the ill child. As with many medical students, I received a print of *The Doctor*, a symbol of professional virtue, as a graduation gift. It hung in my apartments during my residency and at the beginning of my medical career. For the past decades, it has occupied a spot on my office wall. So it may come as a surprise to learn that I have a conflicted relationship with this painting.

Over the years, I've frequently seen this painting in presentations to students and doctors-in-training, most often in talks on professionalism, the duty of the physician, and the art of medicine. The painting is held up as evidence of what's missing in healthcare today: listening and spending time with patients. I applaud the message, but not the mythologizing. Given the challenges facing clinicians today, this idealistic and sensitive framing feels like unfair treatment of a work of art and imposes unrealistic expectations about what needs to be done.

We can't forget that medical science was in its infancy in the latter half of the nineteenth century. Diagnostic testing was limited. Many thought leaders believed miasma, or bad air, was the source of disease. Germ theory was a radical concept. The antibiotic age was fifty years on the horizon. Given the state of medical knowledge and medical practice at that time, physicians had little to offer patients but their presence.

Still, a part of me pines for all that's missing from the scene depicted in *The Doctor*. There are few, if any, of the obstacles that complicate and subvert the connection between doctors and patients. Today, physician productivity estimates suggest 20 to 30 percent of a physician's capacity involves tasks such as documentation, inputting data into the electronic health record, and compliance-related activities. Physicians may spend twice as much time in emergency departments with documentation and duties unrelated to patient care than actual time with patients.

But we should not forget the medical progress accompanying these modern nuisances; advances in diagnostics, treatments, and health systems allow me to provide a level of care unimaginable to physicians centuries ago. Up-to-date knowledge is rapidly accessible with a few clicks or swipes on my computer or smartphone. It's hard to go back to the end of the nineteenth century and pretend such modern advances no longer exist, but *The Doctor* asks how I'd respond if given a choice to trade current knowledge and technology for 30 to 50 percent more time with patients. That is, if I can't have both.

I can't look at Fildes's *The Doctor* now without thinking about these words from Kurt Vonnegut: "We are what we pretend to be, so we must be careful about what we pretend to be."

When technology, business, and political interests have transformed and deformed the practice of medicine, aspiring to a romanticized past strikes me as irresponsible: it's disconnected from modern pressures. For the longest time, *The Doctor* compounded my feelings of inadequacy, a reminder of the meaningful, missing part of my work that, at the same time, feels impossible to reclaim without systemic changes. Caught between two worlds seemingly beyond my control, I felt worse, not better, dogged by defeat from failing to live up to the demands and ideals of both.

Writing a better story for medicine is an endeavor that far exceeds my capacity as a doctor and a writer, but I, along with every other clinician, retain the possibility to write a better story for myself.

The print of *The Doctor* continues to live on my office wall, but not as an object of iconography. Instead, it's a breathing provocation, a reminder that I'm a protagonist in many stories. I think about this painting through my own experiences as a clinician, parent, husband, writer, and patient. Being a passive protagonist won't cut it. I must become an active protagonist, a character willing to struggle through obstacles, beginning with identifying our fears, anxieties, limitations, and various psychic wounds. But what core beliefs are worth fighting for? What are we willing to give up in the process? We don't always find opportunities to consider the different roads we're on—internal and external—and ponder how we want to travel them.

The question "Can you write a better story for yourself" is tied up in the question "What story do you believe you're a part of?" and "Who will you become along the way?"

In 1890, when Sir Henry Tate commissioned a painting from Luke Fildes, he left the painting's subject up to the artist. Luke Fildes drew on a personal tragedy, his son's death at age one from typhoid fever. The "character and bearing of the doctor throughout the time of their anxiety, made a deep impression." I can only imagine the painter's parental anguish at the time, a nightmarish experience out of which this work of art emerged.

Over the years, the enduring power of this work of art, and what I connect to most deeply, is the painter's struggle, his ability to channel his young son's tragic death onto the canvas in a manner that captures a perplexing range of emotions, from worry to grief to hope. I'm drawn more to the background details often missed by those of us who read this work too quickly. The complex, somber tones, haunting images of distraught parents, and the subtle glint of light beyond our attention provide both texture and resistance to the prevailing mood in the scene. I find the sunlight a remarkable detail given Fildes's personal tragedy. It suggests recovery for the young boy, or at least invites the viewer to consider other futures.

The challenges facing clinicians is never-ending. The engine of all stories is the expectation gap between what you expect to happen and what happens. The critical tools for helping patients understand the story of their lives applies to investigations into our own. In my attempts to write a better story for myself, I've discovered it's hard to appreciate an experience without simultaneously, if not unconsciously, comparing it to what you believe it should be.

So, it's okay that *The Doctor* is no longer an inspirational force of idealism for me. It's become so much more. Now it's a friend, a friend with whom I have had a long and intense relationship, someone from whom I expect nothing, only to be there to remind me that the scene is never ideal and our role in it is often conflicted. I've learned from writing that stories aren't always about change but about the possibility of change. We should look for that glint of light in the background shadows, find ways to connect with patients while never losing hold of that person we want to be. Only we can write our own story. And if we're fortunate, the revisions will become our lifelong project.

39
Not an Ending

Mr. Adams complains of chest pressure, some difficulty breathing, and a little sweating. He was afraid he might be having a heart attack. But he's fine now and regrets calling 911. Back to normal? I ask. A little discomfort, he says, but better. Our EKG, which screams heart attack, contradicts his sunny self-assessment. I activate the cardiac catheterization team. The cardiologist on call, one of our finest, makes arrangements to take Mr. Adams immediately to the catheterization (cath) lab. She'll identify the critical blockage starving the damaged part of the heart, thread a stent, and restore blood flow. Dodging severe injury, Mr. Adams will likely go on living his life as before. There's a hitch: Mr. Adams believes he feels too good to be having a heart attack. A catheterization is unnecessary.

When time is muscle and any delay increases the chance of lasting injury, why would Mr. Adams, a generally healthy man in his seventies, deny himself the best possible chance of a good outcome? I talk with him. Listen to his worries, fears, and reasoning. The cardiologist talks with him, too. Did he understand the potentially life-threatening nature of this problem, the benefits and consequences of the various treatment options, including what I soon learned is a desire to be discharged home?

Patients have every right to refuse care, to make decisions, and decide what can and cannot be done with their bodies. I can't distill my frustration with Mr. Adams to concern for his welfare alone. He's not only depriving himself of the best chance to foil a heart attack, he's denying us a pleasure that doesn't come along often—the immediate satisfaction of a good ending.

Early in my career, I was aware of a knock against emergency medicine—a lack of closure. We rarely follow a disease through to the end. We don't see pneumonia improve with antibiotics. We're not tracking the wrist fracture through healing and rehabilitation. Dr. G, a dean at my medical school, a prominent internist and infectious disease researcher, when learning of my intention to enter emergency medicine, said, "Emergency medicine is to internal medicine as the short story is to the novel. And there are no great short story writers."

When Dr. G quipped confidently about the lack of great short story writers, a ticker-tape exploded in my head, silently spitting out names, beginning with Anton Chekhov, who also happened to be a physician.

Whether someone is writing or reading a short story, a long novel, or a poem, the temporal experience will eventually end without necessarily promising closure. *The Oxford English Dictionary* has many definitions for "ending," including termination, conclusion, completion, and death. In the

ER, we're constantly knocking up against endings in these different forms: the end of life; the end of previous expectations of the body and the mind; the end of relationships; the end of compassion; the end of hope; the end of a shift; the sunset of a career.

Endings shouldn't be confused with solutions, though the model of fixing what's broken or controlling what's messy is often the singular acceptable ending in the minds of patients and clinicians. Patients want answers. Insurers tie payment to the diagnosis. By not tagging a label on symptoms or forcing an experience into a specific box, clinicians may fear patients and colleagues will question their diagnostic competence. But such a focus not only disrespects the complex problems and pain endured by our patients, narrowing our focus restricts the openness required to entertain different possibilities, and thus, different endings.

In one respect, every encounter I have with patients ends similarly—with a disposition. Their disposition has nothing to do with their internal character or temperament but their physical destination once they leave the ER. Typically, this means discharge home or admission to the hospital. The disposition for Mr. Adams will be the cath lab, then the cardiac ICU, or the ICU with medical management alone, or leave the ER for home. Regardless, we'll eventually separate and move on. How people move on and my responsibility to them when they're in that other space isn't always clear. We may hold different opinions, doctor and patient. Even two physicians may have different but acceptable visions of a good ending.

Chekhov's stories and plays famously subverted expectations of what an ending should be. He wasn't inclined to moralize or tidy things up at the end. His subversive lack of closure was authentic to the uncertainty of everyday reality. In a letter, Chekhov said, "When I am finished with my characters, I like to return them to life."

Take Tami J, a woman writhing in tears on the stretcher. "I need to have an answer," she begs. Several specialists have evaluated her chronic abdominal pain over the years without identifying a cause for her symptoms. I've learned to accept and interpret such pleas figuratively. Such words are often shorthand for "I can't take this pain anymore" or "You don't understand what it's like to be a young woman who can't go out without fear of the pain flaring up" or "The doctors think I'm crazy and it's all in my head but I'm not crazy—am I?" or "My doctor says I have X, but he doesn't know."

Does she think I'm smarter than all her specialists and their fancy procedures and expertise, that some ER doc, a stranger, has the key to all her troubles? The uncertainty in her situation provides an anchor for next steps, addressing her pain and the conditions that exacerbate or improve her distress. For Tami J, that requires brooding about other medical conditions that might have been missed, chasing down test results, reaching out to her providers, and greasing the gears for timely follow-up. A responsible disposition considers her present suffering and anticipates certain obstacles and challenges that tomorrow might bring. Sure, there is much that is beyond my control, but the impulse to "have an answer" is often satisfied by the tiniest attempts to make the journey of mystery easier.

Which is part of the reason I was apoplectic over Mr. Adams. For all the ways the modern healthcare system falls short, advances in technology have turned acute heart attack and its devastating consequences into a story with a hopeful ending. An excellent catheterization team is gowned up and ready to go. The story is writing itself. Well, that's not precisely accurate. That's the story we're writing. Mr. Adams has other ideas.

I remember Mr. D, an ER patient in his early fifties who, like Mr. Adams, had chest discomfort and suspicious EKG changes and politely refused treatment. He signed out against medical advice despite my urging. I asked the nurse in charge and a social worker to have words with him. I respected them both dearly and hoped they'd find avenues to connect with him. Desperate, I contacted his ex-wife, who wasn't surprised he'd had a heart attack or insisted on leaving without treatment. Mr. D said he knew what he was doing. His father died at his age from a heart attack, uncles as well. He was an avid fisherman and was putting together his rods and gear when the pain started. "You might die, too," I said. He smiled. "I know that," he said, wearing a peaceful expression. "And I'll die catching fish."

Concerning his nuanced and unsettled endings, Virginia Woolf wrote that Chekhov "never manipulates the evidence so as to produce something, fitting, decorous, agreeable to our vanity." My vanity and ego were on display with Mr. Adams. Still, Chekhov offers a potent reminder that the good endings in emergency medicine are not always conventional, observable, or measurable. The desire to force those endings is not only inauthentic to the patient's needs but potentially irresponsible.

The truth is, I'm often conflicted about what makes for a good ending. When we steal from death and bring a patient back to life, I'm often elated. But this feeling of victory is often a false coin. The patient never gets off the ventilator or suffers an anoxic brain injury, and death finally finds her after lingering for days or weeks. What if Mr. Adams, like Mr. D, has visions of his end, his story equivalent of catching fish? I'm responsible for honoring that scene, too. That requires being honest with this moment in his story, even if it resists the urge to be the story we want it to be.

In my writing, I gravitate toward endings that have little to do with closure or solutions. I haven't figured out whether this inclination pushed me into emergency medicine or the uncertainty that saturates my ER practice influenced the type of narratives I find compelling and honest. As a reader, I love finishing a story or essay and carrying the characters, ideas, and challenges in my head when I'm in the car or walking the dog. It relates, I believe, to Chekhov's vision of returning characters to their lives. If I think of my experience with ER patients like a story, then being a responsible physician and writer means thinking about and respecting the patient's life off the page, even if it's chaotic and beyond ordering.

There's provocative research that suggests a connection between readers' self-esteem and their comfort with certain endings. Researchers found participants with lower self-esteem prefer crime or detective stories that confirm their suspicions in the end. Meanwhile, participants with higher self-esteem enjoyed stories that ran against their expectations or the surprise ending. I bring up this research not to implicate readers and their personalities, and not as accepted dogma since my lifetime battle with low self-esteem runs against the authors' findings, but for consideration and reflection: Are there particular endings that make you uneasy? If so, have you thought to ask yourself why?

Patients bring their stories to us and being astute stewards of their stories requires serving as astute gatekeepers of endings.

Mr. Adams, we soon discover, has no family or friends for us to include in or leave out of this discussion. The picture of a lonely man comes into relief. He's not afraid of dying, he says. He's lived a good life, and if it's time to die, he's ready. I share a third narrative future with him, one where he doesn't get better and doesn't die but suffers from a damaged heart. He must leave his apartment and move to a nursing home, where he won't enjoy the independence he relishes now. That's not going to happen, he says.

"How can you be so sure?" I ask, while wondering about how I can be so confident about what I know.

There are many ways to end a story. Whether you're someone who works with words on the page or someone who works with people in ill-fitting gowns—or both—the least we can offer readers, patients, and the people who care for them is a fresh way of looking, an angle into their troubles, a change in perspective that honors their story and their struggles. The novelist E. L. Doctorow gave this now famous advice: "Writing is like driving at night in the fog. You can only see as far as your headlights, but you can make the whole trip that way."

In the ER, where surprises and the unexpected are the norm, I might not have the time, knowledge, or resources to take a full view of a patient's life. But I can catch what's within the arc of a headlight and tend to that. Sometimes that crisis requires life-saving actions. Other times, I'm trying to move their story forward, tend to their uncertainty, pain, and suffering, and make their journey a little smoother or momentarily less lonely. From this perspective, it's easier to locate the possible in the seemingly impossible. The most honest endings move us toward new beginnings.

40
Writing Stories of Medicine

The ground shared between doctors and patients is sacred ground. Privacy laws codify in explicit terms what counts as protected personal information. None of these essays reveal any such details. But there are also moral codes such as respect for privacy and confidentiality that fortify the doctor–patient relationship, and this terrain is trickier to navigate. I altered the names and identifiable details of patients included in these essays. By changing recognizable features, rendering these patients functionally anonymous through descriptive plastic surgery, have I fulfilled my moral responsibility to them?

For years I've worked around my discomfort in this space by using it as inspiration for more imaginative work in my short fiction. The leap into nonfiction required faithfulness to reality, a tether to actual people, and part of the process of learning new skills for this new form of writing also meant confronting my dual and dueling roles as a physician/writer. This book focused on small moments and tensions contained in complex physical and emotional spaces, so I feel an obligation to take you a little deeper into these choppy waters as well.

The teller of stories holds power. The rewards of narrative writing, write journalists Mark Kramer and Wendy Call, are possible only when writers accept ethical responsibility. They acknowledge that a journalist may violate a subject's privacy when gathering material. The journalist Isabel Wilkerson writes, "Narrative writers must strike a careful balance, caring about our subjects without sacrificing our narratives, while caring about our narratives without sacrificing our subjects. . . . Good journalism and empathy can go hand in hand."

As a physician/writer, my first allegiance is to patients and to the moral pillar of trust. Their trust is precious, especially when I'm writing narratives based on clinical experiences where I'm a subject, too. I could have written in abstract or theoretical terms, but it would lose specificity, immediacy, and urgency. It would cease being a narrative.

My duty as a writer is to be sensitive to this tension, heed its pull, and be as responsible as possible. In practical terms, this means continually evaluating which details belong solely to the physician or the patient, what information might be considered shared custody, and what elements should be left off the table entirely because they're too intimate or fragile or because they're not foundational to the story.

Such dissection isn't easy or perfect. Only rarely am I compelled to write about a specific clinical interaction. But when similar types of experiences keep arising, either my own or those of colleagues, it tugs on my sleeve. A particular case may anchor a piece of writing. But through the process of writing and rewriting, I'll interrogate and weigh and scrub at details. I'll ask myself: What are you trying to say, and what elements are necessary to further that discussion? What can be left out or changed entirely to protect patient privacy? I test the architecture of faithfulness to a particular situation while striving for a certain universality. I'll put it this way: if I've done my job well, there might be three or five or ten patients and physicians who could mistakenly see themselves in one of these essays.

Why didn't I get the patient's consent? The consent process is muddied because I never care for patients with my writer's hat. The physician/writer must be first, and foremost, a physician. I never know what sticks with me and why and how or if I'll use it later. Typically, many years pass before an experience finds its way into a narrative. I don't keep track of patients' names because I'm not thinking of them as narrative subjects. It's also protected health information.

William Carlos Williams said his medical badge "was the thing which gained me entrance to those secret gardens of the self."

The physician/writer must be ever sensitive to the moral landmines when writing emerges from experiences with patients. We can never forget that certain bedside obligations carry forward into our writing, including respect, honesty, trustworthiness, and compassion. Altering identifiable details isn't enough. Being a morally responsible and accountable physician/writer requires imagination. I pretend the patient is looking over my shoulder as I write. Would they consider the writing fair, thoughtful, responsible, the best it could be? And, would they still respect me as a physician?

41
One Last Thing

When I delivered the completed manuscript to my editor in April 2021, the COVID-19 pandemic was just beginning to release its tight squeeze on our lives. Experts opined about a return to normalcy, and that possibility couldn't come soon enough. Working in the ER through two waves of the pandemic left me feeling like an odd-textured human—crispy on the outside and committed, yet disillusioned and slightly raw on the inside. And I wasn't alone. A national survey at that time noted six in ten healthcare workers said the stress from the pandemic harmed their mental health, and three in ten considered leaving their profession.

Luckily, as this book's manuscript left my hands, researchers had developed vaccines in record time, pharmaceutical companies had moved them to market, and leaders were rallying (or stumbling) to get them into people's arms. Spring was here, too, bringing the warm kiss of sunlight on my unmasked face and hugs with friends and family whom I hadn't seen in quite a while. The 2021 forecast called for a summer of hope. I couldn't wait for a reunion with pre-COVID-19 problems and health system hiccups.

As many of you know too well, the COVID-19 delta variant had other plans, and the summer of hope descended us into yet another crisis. Many people weren't rushing to get vaccinated; facial coverings, social distancing, and public health measures were ignored if not overtly rebuffed. The public cries of resistance, grounded in self-interest, individual liberties, misinformation, or mistrust, resulted in record numbers of COVID-19 cases and deaths. Meanwhile, pleas and thunder from the media and digital platforms such as Twitter for the unvaccinated to get the vaccine—often spiced with caps, exclamation points, and emoji—wasn't promoting trust, empathy, and behavior change. The polarizing public discourse felt as lethal as any novel virus.

As this book goes through final edits in October 2021, only 66 percent of the population in the United States have received a dose of one of the COVID-19 vaccines. But from my work as a clinician and a writer, I know there's unstable ground beneath hard data, data-defying mysteries playing out in individual lives, a narrative crisis complicating the life-saving efforts of leaders in infectious disease and public health.

Mustering sympathy for the unvaccinated was hard, especially when I cared for too many people who might not be sick from COVID-19 or struggling for their lives had they only been vaccinated. However, in my anger appeared pools of sorrow. The unvaccinated weren't all defiant. By way of an explanation, I'd often get a shrug or a look of confusion, which left me feeling confused and a little seasick. These individuals didn't know what to believe when truth itself has supply-chain problems, and the healthcare system has been letting them down for years. While I agreed with the voices who called out those who didn't take precautions to protect their health and safeguard the well-being of others as irresponsible, I quickly recognized that throwing all the unvaccinated into the same whirlpool of blame was irresponsible as well.

This tension bothered me. To objectify my thinking and work through these competing realities, I began writing. I found myself arguing for something so basic and unimpressive—reasonable and open discourse—that I stopped multiple times. I can't be writing something so obvious? Then I'd open Twitter or follow my Apple News feed and end up back at my desk. The echo chambers on the extreme right and left were creating firestorms, not engagement and connection. They smothered the voices who made camp in the messy middle, a lost and lonely outpost where thinking in nuance and trading in shades of gray aren't readily heard.

The small piece was published in *STAT* on August 27, 2021. The response surprised and destabilized me in profound and not entirely pleasant ways. The overwhelmingly positive response, the comments that a call for reason was somehow an act of bravery, startled me. As were the impressively insulting trolls who had no interest in civility or punctuation.

The reader feedback I cherished the most came from unvaccinated people who wanted to discuss why they were hesitant. Someone didn't have a doctor or someone in the healthcare profession she trusted for advice. Even so, she wears a mask, socially distances, and does her best to be responsible to herself and others. One person described searching the internet and not knowing what or who to believe. Several readers hated being labeled as "anti-vax" or "selfish." One person said she got a flu shot every year. She didn't have a problem with vaccines that have been well studied, only the COVID vaccine. Another person echoed a common theme: a lack of trust in the vaccine development process, drawing on credibility problems with pharmaceutical companies, including a history of data manipulation and fraud. I was surprised they packaged the new cutting-edge mRNA vaccine as "Operation Warp Speed," an almost comically tone-deaf name that doesn't soothe those who are wary of the integrity of the science and the research trials. Readers shared their doubts about governmental agencies such as the CDC and FDA. One person summed up their bind: they either trust their competency and integrity or do not, and should they not, they get labeled as dangerous by those who do. They weren't screaming, but carefully explaining the sources of their doubt and the many sides of their stories.

No single narrative can hold the weight of this moment and the decisions people must make when faced with high-stakes uncertainty and different frames of belief. I received pushback from people I adore and respect, including many colleagues I work with, who I figured would appreciate a voice from the messy middle. Instead, a common remark was: Yeah, I read your piece. But the unvaccinated need to get the #%$ing shot (add adjective of choice). My favorite came from a former emergency medicine resident, a mentee with whom I'm very close. She said, "I agree with you, Baruch. But I still want to punch you in the face."

I get it. This time around, the crisis was avoidable. One can only speculate the outcome if enough people had taken the necessary precautions, including getting the vaccine. Would hospitals still be inundated with sick patients— COVID-19 and otherwise—and struggling to meet the most basic levels of clinical excellence, efficiency, and compassion? The waiting times are orders of magnitude greater than the pre-COVID-19 wait times I write about in this book. Certain states implemented crisis standards of care policies, which are activated when hospitals face resource shortages that "place a patient or provider at risk of a poor outcome." Some overwhelmed hospitals transferred patients to open beds in ICUs in different parts of the country, far from family and friends.

Close to home, my moral tank was leaking. Erecting a protective shell allowed me to stay afloat but at the expense of feeling less. But absorbing the full impact of the conditions of care and the unmet needs of patients broke my heart. Either way, each ER shift produced a few more psychic paper cuts, and I tried not to make a mess. My colleagues confided in me their experiences of moral injury and emotional and physical exhaustion. Soon, teary goodbyes with another nurse, physician, or staff member became another part of this ongoing story.

The efforts from clinicians, researchers, and experts from many disciplines to understand this novel virus, trace how it moves and operates in the world and our bodies, and then develop a vaccine to protect us against it, were a herculean accomplishment. But this achievement pales next to the problems exposed and amplified by the pandemic that has been with us for years. How do we become knowable, relatable, and responsible to one another in a world that's fraught with uncertainty and doubt and forces seemingly beyond our control?

Is it even possible? Focusing on stories, the smallest stories, might be our only way to move forward together.

Stories reveal how people face, cope, succumb, and surmount the obstacles in their lives and make their way in a world we all share. They serve as portals of social interaction that pipe us emotionally into the experience of another. That can't happen unless we lower our guard, draw up our courage, and invite people into our lives, even if it's only a few steps. And when the door creaks open, we must find the courage to take those steps. Stories are more powerful than data. To persuade people, to get them to think, you must first get them to understand that you care.

Sometimes there's anger. Frustration perhaps. And sadness, and maybe a hint of empathy. If we're lucky, there's humor, too. What's better than an unexpected, shared laugh as a shortcut to connection? Ideally, we'll feel all these emotions and many more. That's okay. Stories can hold them, especially when built on shared islands of trust. Respectful disagreement begins with openness and curiosity and the willingness to seek out common values and experiences.

Caring for patients begins with caring for their stories. If I've learned anything in my three decades as a professional listener and teller of stories, in the ER and on the page, it is the importance of humility. We humans are beautifully flawed creatures with inexplicable needs and impulses that often run counter to our best interests. As this book illustrates, it's not always easy to understand another human, but it's possible and necessary. We're not going to be perfect, but making this effort matters, especially now, because we must find a way to rise to the occasion, together.

Acknowledgments

This acknowledgment section is my attempt to express gratitude and fallibility. The people and work whose influence directly or indirectly permeate the book are so vast and profound, I'll invariably omit essential people in the few pages I have. So, to those inspiring individuals, thank you.

This book reflects ideas that bridge medicine, humanities, writing, and the creative arts. The opportunity to pursue this type of interdisciplinary exploration would never have happened without the encouragement of key people across Brown University, starting with Brian Zink, my former chairman in the Department of Emergency Medicine, Alpert Medical School at Brown University. Michael Steinberg, the former director of the Cogut Institute for the Humanities at Brown University, provided an emergency physician an opportunity as a faculty fellow at the Cogut Institute in spring 2011, and the staff had provided a home away from home for a decade. For several special years, Ian Gonsher and a remarkable ragtag group of faculty and students pushed my thinking in the Creative Scholars Project at the Granoff Center for the Arts at Brown University.

Many of these essays were previously published in different forms. The published pieces were infinitely better than what first appeared in the editors' inboxes. I'm forever grateful to *STAT* First Opinion editor Pat Skerrett, who nudged me to write clearer, sharper, and tighter prose. I also learned from pieces that he politely rejected with "next time." This book wouldn't have found the attention of the MIT Press without *STAT* and their encouragement and reach as a platform.

A few essays appeared on WBUR's *Cognoscenti* after passing through the keen editorial eyes of editors Frannie Carr Toth and Cloe Axelson. Some first appeared in *Hastings Center Report*, a publication from one of the oldest and widely respected bioethics centers. I've always considered ethical dilemmas as critical moments in a story, so the opportunity to appear in their pages was always a thrill. I want to acknowledge the editors at the *New England Journal of Medicine*, the *Health Humanities Reader* (Rutgers University Press), and the *Annals of Internal Medicine*.

This book is the culmination of over a decade of thinking and teaching, giving visiting lectures, and working on a range of projects. Thank you to friends and colleagues at the American Society for Bioethics and Humanities and the American College of Emergency Physician Medical Humanities sub-section; Kirsten Ostherr and Bryan Vartabedian, who years ago invited me to Baylor University and the Medical Futures Labs conference to talk about story and narrative at a meeting centered on technology and the future of medicine; Ronan Kavanagh, who welcomed me to Dublin to work through some ideas about "not-knowing" at dotMD and the inspiring community of dotMD friends.

I've been fortunate to teach and write and intersect with so many extraordinary people. They include Kelli Auerbach, Christine Montross, Michael Barthman, Stacey Springs, Kevin Liou, Marty Kohn, Jack Coulehan, Stephanie Brown Clark, Arno Kumagai, Katie Watson, Art Derse, Gretchen Case, Delese Wear, Joyce Rosenfeld, Tess Jones, Erin Lamb, Pam Schaff, Kathryn Montgomery, Arthur Frank, Resa Lewiss, Amy Haddad, Rita Charon, Nellie Hermann, Ash Adam, Tonya Waldburger, John de Szendeffy, Hollis Mickey, Alexandra Poterack, Sarah Ganz Blythe, Fred Schiffman, and on and on. Over the years, I've had the good fortune to cross paths and collaborate with incredible people on the other side of the hill at the Rhode Island School of Design. Specifically, I want to acknowledge the Center for Complexity and the museum educators at the Rhode Island School of Design Museum.

I owe a huge debt of gratitude to Mikkael Sekeres, a friend, physician, and writer I admire greatly.

This book wouldn't be possible without Bob Prior, my editor at the MIT Press, who deftly handled the words and psyche of a writer who was working ER shifts during three waves of a pandemic. I also want to express my deepest gratitude to Judith Feldmann for her patience and guidance through the copyediting process, the incredible designer Yasuyo Iguchi, and the amazing publicity and marketing team headed by Nicholas DiSabatino and Jessica Pellien, including Corrine Gould, Matt Badessa, Anar Badalov, Rachel Aldrich, and Lissa Warren. To the staff at MIT Press, thank you for being so wonderful, especially when you were challenged by the pandemic, too.

I've been lucky to work in the Department of Emergency Medicine at Alpert Medical School at Brown University, a place rich with talented, caring clinicians—faculty and residents—who are also experts in a wide range of disciplines. My thinking has been inspired and sharpened by bouncing against these people whose interests and academic work is often very different from my own. They're also compassionate and funny. Thank you to the nurses, advanced practice providers, ER staff, residents, and colleagues in other departments, and to patients and families for teaching me so much. A big thanks to the passionate medical educators at Alpert Medical School and the gift of mentoring and learning from an extraordinary group of medical students.

To my sister Amy, sounding board, fellow ER doc, sharp reader, and great cook, and to my niece Michelle; and to my parents, Mel and Lucy Baruch—I'm forever thankful and lucky to share love and DNA.

This book, ultimately, belongs to my wife Jen, for her love and patience and unapologetic but necessary feedback on the manuscript; and to my son Daniel, who possesses an intelligence and warmth that make a father proud. My family had to put up with the crazy COVID world while living with a nutty ER doc writing a book. Lucky for me, they're crazy, too. And very funny. My family. Love you.

Several essays were previously published, often in different forms with different titles. I want to acknowledge and thank the editors and publishers.

STAT

"I'm an Ambassador to Nightmares. My Medical Training Didn't Prepare Me for That"

"Did I Just Feed an Addiction? Or Ease a Man's Pain? Welcome to Modern Medicine's Moral Cage Fight"

"When Death Is Imminent, End-of-Life Decisions Sometimes Go Out the Window"

"Caring for the Caregiver in the Emergency Department"

"On a Frigid Night, Do I Let a Homeless Patient Keep an ER Bed or Free It Up for Someone Who May Need It More?"

"When Waiting Feels Immoral: Fairness in the ER Calls for Empathy from All of Us"

"'Stuck in the Tornado of Life': A Patient's Chaos Narrative"

"When Loneliness Is an Emergency"

"Abandoned by U.S. Leaders, the Only COVID-19 Protection I Can Count on in My Emergency Department Is Trust"

"You Are Waiting for the Surge"

"As a Doctor in the COVID-19 Era, I've Learned That Judging Patients' Decisions Comes Easier Than It Should"

"It's Easy to Judge the Unvaccinated. As a Doctor, I See a Better Alternative"

The Hastings Center Report

"Dr. Douchebag: A Tale of the ER"

"Hug, or Ugh"

"Benefit Paradox"

"Why Won't My Patient Act Like a Jerk"

Cognoscienti

"The Patient Who Said She Wanted Nothing"

"To Talk about Guns, We Must Start with a Grieving Mother's Silence"

"Loving an Old Dog, and Knowing When to Let Him Go"

The Health Humanities Reader, Rutgers University Press

"In Defense of Cheaper Stethoscopes"

Annals of Internal Medicine

"Big Incision"

New England Journal of Medicine

"When Sensitivity Is a Liability"

Notes

2 Not the Beginning

Rebecca Solnit writes, "The word emergency comes from emerge, to rise out of . . .": Rebecca Solnit, *A Paradise Built in Hell* (New York: Penguin Books, 2009).

My work as an emergency physician has always struck me as a fundamentally creative act: Jay Baruch, "Doctors as Makers," *Academic Medicine* 92 (2017): 40–44.

The medical encounter has been compared to improvisation: Katie Watson, "Perspective: Serious Play: Teaching Medical Skills with Improvisational Theater Techniques," *Academic Medicine* 86, no. 10 (2011): 1260–1265; Paul Haidet, "Jazz and the 'Art' of Medicine: Improvisation in the Medical Encounter," *Annals of Family Medicine* 5, no. 2 (March 20072): 164–169.

Our brains are hardwired for story, and the story we create may be very different from the one a patient is telling: Jonathan Gottschall, *The Storytelling Animal: How Stories Make Us Human* (Boston: Houghton Mifflin Harcourt, 2012); Lisa Cron, *Wired for Story* (Berkeley: Ten Speed Press, 2012).

there are only three principal elements to memorize: character, desire, and conflict: Robert McKee, *Story: Substance, Structure, Style and the Principles of Screenwriting* (New York: ReganBooks, 1997).

the tension between seemingly misfit pieces is a fertile place . . . : Charles Baxter, "On Defamiliarization," in *Burning Down the House* (St. Paul, MN: Graywolf Press, 2008).

3   Tornado of Life

the ER: "Emergency room" (ER) is a term that persists from the 1950s when the ER was a single room. As the specialty of emergency medicine has evolved, the ER has expanded into major departments in modern hospitals encompassing many, many rooms. The proper language is now "emergency department." However, the term ER is still commonly used. (Besides, ED has become synonymous with erectile dysfunction.) For the sake of simplicity and consistency, we will use the abbreviation ER, though there are places when you'll see the term "emergency department."

The sociologist Arthur Frank framed the pivotal idea of chaos narratives, and "To deny a chaos story is to deny the person telling the story": Arthur Frank, *The Wounded Storyteller: Body, Illness and Ethics* (Chicago: University of Chicago Press, 1997). I'm grateful to Arthur Frank for his conceptual work that not only informed this story, but seeped into my career caring for patients.

Quest stories borrow from the work of Joseph Campbell: Joseph Campbell, *The Hero with a Thousand Faces* (Princeton, NJ: Princeton University Press, 1973).

4   Backstory

The EMS (emergency medical services): EMS stands for emergency medical services. It's a broad term that includes all first responders. I will be using EMS to denote the prehospital providers, including paramedics and EMTs, for this book. Though these terms are widely known, they represent various levels and scope of training. For example, there are several levels of training for EMTs (basic, advanced, cardiac, and paramedic), and names are often used interchangeably in a manner that may be confusing. To minimize that, and out of respect and appreciation for the incredible work of all our prehospital colleagues, I'll use EMS more broadly. (Thanks to Dr. Nick Asselin and my Brown EMS Division faculty for their input.)

"Clinicians . . . work to perfect the map of illness, but each patient, each instance of illness, is unchartered territory": Kathryn Montgomery Hunter, *Doctors' Stories: The Narrative Structure of Medical Knowledge* (Princeton, NJ: Princeton University Press, 1991).

5   Why Medicine Needs More Not-Knowing

"Landscapes can be deceptive . . .": John Berger, *A Fortunate Man* (New York: Vintage, 1997).

In this essay, Barthelme describes the act of writing, and the creative arts in general . . . : Donald Barthelme and Kim A. Herzinger, *Not-Knowing: The Essays and Interviews of Donald Barthelme* (New York: Random House, 1997).

"Absolute certainty in diagnosis is unattainable . . .": Jerome P. Kassirer, "Our Stubborn Quest for Diagnostic Certainty," *New England Journal of Medicine* 320, no. 22 (1989): 1489–1491.

A study reported that 75 clinical trials and 11 systematic reviews are published each day: H. Bastian, P. Glasziou, and I. Chalmers, "Seventy-Five Trials and Eleven Systematic Reviews a Day: How Will We Ever Keep Up?" *PLOS Medicine* 7, no. 9 (2010).

When writing stories, you move into what Eudora Welty calls "open spaces": Eudora Welty, *The Eye of the Story* (New York. Vintage International, 1993).

Narrative is an "invitation to problem finding, not a lesson in problem solving": Jerome Bruner, *Actual Minds, Possible Worlds* (Cambridge, MA: Harvard University Press, 1987); Jerome Bruner, *Making Stories: Law, Literature and Life* (Cambridge, MA: Harvard University Press, 2002).

"in any process of inquiry, our uncertainty is our ally": Mark Doty, "In Favor of Uncertainty," in *Views from the Loft*, edited by Daniel Slager (Minneapolis: Milkweed Editions, 2010).

6   Ambassador to Nightmares

Studies show the public is overly optimistic when it comes to predicting recovery after cardiopulmonary resuscitation: G. K. Jones, K. L. Brewer, and H. G. Garrison, "Public Expectations of Survival Following Cardiopulmonary Resuscitation," *Academic Emergency Medicine* 7, no. 1 (2000): 48–53.

The media contributes to the misinformation: J. J. Van den Bulck, "The Impact of Television Fiction on Public Expectations of Survival Following

Inhospital Cardiopulmonary Resuscitation by Medical Professionals," *European Journal of Emergency Medicine* 9, no. 4 (2002): 325–329.

People on television shows whose hearts stop recover more often than in real life: S. J. Diem, J. D. Lantos, and J. A. Tulsky, "Cardiopulmonary Resuscitation on Television. Miracles and Misinformation," *New England Journal of Medicine* 334, no. 24 (1996): 1578–1582.

Death from trauma such as car crashes . . . : A. E. Stewart, "Complicated Bereavement and Posttraumatic Stress Disorder Following Fatal Car Crashes: Recommendations for Death Notification Practice," *Death Studies* 23, no. 4 (1999): 289–321.

That wasn't uncommon at the time: A. M. Sullivan, A. G. Warren, M. D. Lakoma, K. R. Liaw, D. Hwang, and S. D. Block, "End-of-Life Care in the Curriculum: A National Study of Medical Education Deans," *Academic Medicine* 79, no. 8 (2004): 760–768.

Despite the best efforts to study, understand, and train for these encounters: Jan M. Shoenberger, Sevan Yeghiazarian, Claritza Rios, and Sean O. Henderson, "Death Notification in the Emergency Department: Survivors and Physicians," *Western Journal of Emergency Medicine* 14, no. 2 (2013): 181; Cherri Hobgood, Donna Harward, Kelly Newton, and William Davis, "The Educational Intervention 'GRIEV_ING' Improves the Death Notification Skills of Residents," *Academic Emergency Medicine* 12, no. 4 (2005): 296–301; Kenneth V. Iserson, "Topic in Review: Notifying Survivors about Sudden, Unexpected Deaths," *Western Journal of Medicine* 173, no. 4 (2000): 261; Terri A. Schmidt, Robert L. Norton, and Susan W. Tolle, "Sudden Death in the Ed: Educating Residents to Compassionately Inform Families," *Journal of Emergency Medicine* 10, no. 5 (1992): 643–647.

Families remember these moments: Sharon Roman, "Breaking Bad News—Find a Way to Bridge the Gap," *British Medical Journal* (2017), published electronically August 2, 2017, https://blogs.bmj.com/bmj/2017/08/02/sharon-roman-breaking-bad-news-find-a-way-to-bridge-the-gap/; M. Schmid Mast, A. Kindlimann, and W. Langewitz, "Recipients' Perspective on Breaking Bad News: How You Put It Really Makes a Difference," *Patient Education and Counseling* 58, no. 3 (Sep 2005): 244–251.

In situations like these, the family members become victims themselves . . . : R. Zalenski, R. F. Gillum, T. E. Quest, and J. L. Griffith, "Care for the Adult Family Members of Victims of Unexpected Cardiac Death," *Academic Emergency Medicine* 13, no. 12 (2006): 1333–1338.

A seventy-eight-year-old patient with chronic lung disease and difficulty breathing . . . : Julia Jacobs, "Doctor on Video Screen Told a Man He Was Near Death, Leaving Relatives Aghast," *New York Times* (2019), published electronically March 9, 2019, https://www.nytimes.com/2019/03/09/science/telemedicine-ethical-issues.html.

8   When Loneliness Is an Emergency

Iona is the protagonist in Anton Chekhov's 1886 short story "Misery": Anton Chekhov, *Early Short Stories 1883–1888*, translated by Constance Garnett (Modern Library, 1999).

Approximately one in three older Americans report feeling lonely: AARP Foundation, *Loneliness and Social Connections: A National Survey of Adults 45 and Older* (2018).

A review found that individuals without meaningful social relationships are twice as likely to die: J. Holt-Lunstad, T. B. Smith, and J. B. Layton, "Social Relationships and Mortality Risk: A Meta-analytic Review," *PLOS Medicine* 7, no. 7 (2010): e1000316, https://doi.org/10.1371/journal.pmed.1000316; J. Holt-Lunstad, T. B. Smith, M. Baker, T. Harris, and D. Stephenson, "Loneliness and Social Isolation as Risk Factors for Mortality: A Meta-Analytic Review," *Perspectives on Psychological Science* 10, no. 2 (2015): 227–237; R. Rubin, "Loneliness Might Be a Killer, but What's the Best Way to Protect against It?" *JAMA* 318, no. 19 (2017): 1853–1855.

In the UK, the government went so far as to appoint a Minister of Loneliness: Nicholas Pimlott, "The Ministry of Loneliness," *Canadian Family Physician* 64 (2018): 166–166.

It's hard to admit to loneliness: Vivek Murthy, *Together: The Healing Power of Human Connection in a Sometimes Lonely World* (New York: HarperCollins, 2020).

Emergency departments shoulder the acute care burden for insured and uninsured populations: Kristy Gonzalez Morganti, Sebastian Bauhoff, Janice C. Blanchard, Mahshid Abir, Neema Iyer, Alexandria Smith, Joseph

Vesely, Edward N. Okeke, and Arthur L. Kellermann, *The Evolving Role of Emergency Departments in the United States* (RAND Corporation, 2013).

"To look is an act of choice": John Berger, *Ways of Seeing* (New York: Penguin Books, 1972).

Or, would I interrupt him, as studies found, at around twenty-three seconds? M. K. Marvel, R. M. Epstein, K. Flowers, and H. B. Beckman, "Soliciting the Patient's Agenda: Have We Improved?" *JAMA* 281, no. 3 (Jan 20 1999): 283–287; Howard B. Beckman and Richard M. Frankel, "The Effect of Physician Behavior on the Collection of Data," *Annals of Internal Medicine* 101, no. 5 (1984): 692–696; Larry B. Mauksch, "Questioning a Taboo: Physicians' Interruptions During Interactions with Patients," *JAMA* 317, no. 10 (2017): 1021–1022.

Dr. John Lantos has written about how we see ourselves more easily in stories: John Lantos, "Why Doctors Make Good Protagonists," in *Walker Percy and the Moral Life of Medicine*, edited by John Lantos Carl Elliot (Durham: Duke University Press, 1999).

10   Upside Down

"We must look for centers of simplicity in homes with many rooms . . .": Gaston Bachelard, *The Poetics of Space* (New York: Penguin Books, 2014).

12   Narrative Risks: Shape, Place, and Gutter

In a 1944 social psychology study . . . : Fritz Heider and Marianne Simmel, "An Experimental Study of Apparent Behavior," *American Journal of Psychology* 57, no. 2 (1944): 243–259.

Lev Kuleshov, a Russian filmmaker: Marta Calbi, Katrin Heimann, Daniel Barratt, Francesca Siri, Maria A Umiltà, and Vittorio Gallese, "How Context Influences Our Perception of Emotional Faces: A Behavioral Study on the Kuleshov Effect," *Frontiers in Psychology* 8 (2017): 1684.

Scott McLoud describes gutters: Scott McCloud, *Making Comics* (New York: HarperCollins, 2006). Many years ago, this book influenced my thinking about the relationship between image, language, gutters, and the reader's role in constructed stories. It pushed me to think differently about the clinical encounter.

Our brains' craving for narrative coherence: Jonathan Gottschall, *The Storytelling Animal: How Stories Make Us Human* (Boston: Houghton Mifflin Harcourt, 2012).

Kahneman writes how our mind is predisposed to jump to conclusions: Daniel Kahneman, *Thinking, Fast and Slow* (New York: Farrar, Straus and Giroux, 2011).

14 Hug, or Ugh

Research shows that people with traits of extroversion such as sociability and spontaneity are your prototypical huggers: L. M. Forsell and J. A. Åström, "Meanings of Hugging: From Greeting Behavior to Touching Implications," *Comprehensive Psychology* (January 2012); Melissa Locker, "Why Some People Hate Being Hugged, According to Science," *Time*, September 4, 2018, https://time.com/5379586/people-hate-hugged-science/.

An argument can be made that a hug deserves recognition as a bona fide medical treatment: Kathleen C. Light, Karen M. Grewen, and Janet A. Amico, "More Frequent Partner Hugs and Higher Oxytocin Levels Are Linked to Lower Blood Pressure and Heart Rate in Premenopausal Women," *Biological Psychology* 69, no. 1 (2005): 5–21; Sheldon Cohen, Denise Janicki-Deverts, Ronald B. Turner, and William J. Doyle, "Does Hugging Provide Stress-Buffering Social Support? A Study of Susceptibility to Upper Respiratory Infection and Illness," *Psychological Science* 26, no. 2 (2015): 135–147; Michael L. M. Murphy, Denise Janicki-Deverts, and Sheldon Cohen, "Receiving a Hug Is Associated with the Attenuation of Negative Mood That Occurs on Days with Interpersonal Conflict," *PLOS ONE* 13, no. 10 (2018): e0203522.

In the United States and other countries, there's a National Hugging Day: "National Hugging Day," official website, https://www.nationalhugging day.com.

15 Moving On

When physicians suffer, patients may suffer, too: D. W. Lu, S. Dresden, C. McCloskey, J. Branzetti, and M. A. Gisondi, "Impact of Burnout on Self-Reported Patient Care among Emergency Physicians," *Western Journal of Emergency Medicine* 16, no. 7 (Dec 2015): 996–1001.

Many influences contribute to burnout in medicine: T. D. Shanafelt, "Enhancing Meaning in Work: A Prescription for Preventing Physician Burnout and Promoting Patient-Centered Care," *JAMA* 302, no. 12 (2009): 1338–1340, https://doi.org/10.1001/jama.2009.1385.

There are stressors specific to emergency medicine that place its practitioners at further risk for burnout: Eric Berger, "Physician Burnout," *Annals of Emergency Medicine* 3, no. 61 (2013): A17–A19.

16   Compassion at the Crossroads

The crisis of emergency department crowding: C. Morley, M. Unwin, G. M. Peterson, J. Stankovich, and L. Kinsman, "Emergency Department Crowding: A Systematic Review of Causes, Consequences and Solutions," *PLOS ONE* 13, no. 8 (2018): e0203316.

Crowding and prolonged waits in the ER [are] linked to grave medical consequences:

higher inpatient mortality: B. C. Sun, R. Y. Hsia, R. E. Weiss, D. Zingmond, L. J. Liang, W. Han, H. McCreath, and S. M. Asch, "Effect of Emergency Department Crowding on Outcomes of Admitted Patients," *Annals of Emergency Medicine* 61, no. 6 (2013): 605–611.

longer length of stay in the hospital: Adam J. Singer, Henry C. Thode Jr., Peter Viccellio, and Jesse M. Pines, "The Association between Length of Emergency Department Boarding and Mortality," *Academic Emergency Medicine* 18, no. 12 (2011): 1324–1329.

more harmful cardiac outcomes: Jesse M. Pines, Charles V. Pollack Jr., Deborah B. Diercks, Anna Marie Chang, Frances S Shofer, and Judd E Hollander, "The Association between Emergency Department Crowding and Adverse Cardiovascular Outcomes in Patients with Chest Pain," *Academic Emergency Medicine* 16, no. 7 (2009): 617–625.

delayed treatment for pain: Angela M. Mills, Frances S. Shofer, Esther H. Chen, Judd E. Hollander, and Jesse M. Pines, "The Association between Emergency Department Crowding and Analgesia Administration in Acute Abdominal Pain Patients," *Academic Emergency Medicine* 16, no. 7 (2009): 603–608.

Severe mental illness afflicts up to a quarter of all homeless people: Rebecca Sturgis, Adam Sirgany, Michael Stoops, and Neil J Donovan, *Mental Illness and Homelessness* (National Coaltion for the Homeless, 2010).

Hypothermia is a preventable tragedy: Jeffrey Berko, Deborah D. Ingram, Shubhayu Saha, Jennifer D. Parker, *Deaths Attributed to Heat, Cold, and Other Weather Events in the United States, 2006–2010* (Hyattsville, MD: Centers for Disease Control and Prevention National Center for Health Statistics, 2014).

17   Pain: A Story That's Hard to Treat

data from the CDC show that four out of five heroin users began their habit by using prescription opioids: Nora D. Volkow and A. Thomas McLellan, "Opioid Abuse in Chronic Pain—Misconceptions and Mitigation Strategies," *New England Journal of Medicine* 374, no. 13 (2016): 1253–1263; Rose A. Rudd, Noah Aleshire, Jon E. Zibbell, R. Matthew Gladden, "Increases in Drug and Opioid Overdose Deaths—United States, 2000–2014," *Morbidity and Mortality Weekly Report* 64, no. 50 (2016): 1378–1382.

Prescribing guidelines from the Centers for Disease Control and Prevention: Deborah Dowell, Tamara M. Haegerich, and Roger Chou, "CDC Guideline for Prescribing Opioids for Chronic Pain—United States, 2016," *JAMA* 315, no. 15 (2016): 1624–1645.

The physician/writer David Biro writes achingly about pain: David Biro, *The Language of Pain: Finding Words, Compassion, and Relief* (New York: W. W. Norton, 2010).

In her book The Body in Pain, Elaine Scarry says it best: "To have pain is to have certainty; to hear about pain is to have doubt." Elaine Scarry, *The Body in Pain: The Making and Unmaking of the World* (New York: Oxford University Press, 1987).

the Joint Commission wed farce with policy and declared pain a fifth vital sign . . . : Kristina Fiore, "Opioid Crisis: Scrap Pain as 5th Vital Sign?" *MedPage*, 2016, https://www.medpagetoday.com/publichealthpolicy/publichealth /57336. The Joint Commision is the "oldest and largest standards-setting and accrediting body in health care." For more information, see the

organization's website, https://www.jointcommission.org/about-us/facts
-about-the-joint-commission/joint-commission-faqs/.

Decades of experience have created an internal radar for red-flag behaviors: Randy A. Sansone and Lori A Sansone, "Doctor Shopping: A Phenomenon of Many Themes," *Innovations in Clinical Neuroscience* 9, nos. 11–12 (2012): 42.

A good story engages our emotions and slips past our analytical neural circuitry: Maria Konnikova, *The Confidence Game* (New York: Penguin Books, 2017).

In fact, a coupling develops between the speaker and listener, creating a synchronized neural activity: G. J. Stephens, L. J. Silbert, and U. Hasson, "Speaker–Listener Neural Coupling Underlies Successful Communication," *Proceedings of the National Academy of Sciences* 107, no. 32 (2010): 14425–14430.

Once transported in this way, there's a tendency: Melanie C. Green and Timothy C. Brock, "The Role of Transportation in the Persuasiveness of Public Narratives," *Journal of Personality and Social Psychology* 79, no. 5 (2000): 701–721.

A well-told story with a dramatic arc can elicit empathy: J. A. Barraza, V. Alexander, L. E. Beavin, E. T. Terris, and P. J. Zak, "The Heart of the Story: Peripheral Physiology During Narrative Exposure Predicts Charitable Giving," *Biological Psychology* 105 (Feb. 2015): 138–143.

Patients with sickle cell disease endure severe pain: Paula Tanabe, Randall Myers, Amy Zosel, Jane Brice, Altaf H. Ansari, Julia Evans, Zoran Martinovich, Knox H. Todd, and Judith A. Paice, "Emergency Department Management of Acute Pain Episodes in Sickle Cell Disease," *Academic Emergency Medicine* 14, no. 5 (2007): 419–425; Beryl Lieff Benderly, "Fighting Painful Misconceptions about Sickle Cell Disease in the ER," *Kaiser Health News*, January 24, 2013, https://khn.org/news/sickle-cell-misconceptions-and-the-er/.

Blacks and Hispanics are more likely than non-whites to receive no analgesia: Knox H. Todd, Christi Deaton, Anne P. D'Adamo, and Leon Goe, "Ethnicity and Analgesic Practice," *Annals of Emergency Medicine* 35, no.

1 (2000): 11–16; Knox H. Todd, Nigel Samaroo, and Jerome R. Hoffman, "Ethnicity as a Risk Factor for Inadequate Emergency Department Analgesia," *JAMA* 269, no. 12 (1993): 1537–1539.

Studies show racial and ethnic disparities in opioid prescribing: Joshua H. Tamayo-Sarver, Susan W. Hinze, Rita K. Cydulka, and David W. Baker, "Racial and Ethnic Disparities in Emergency Department Analgesic Prescription," *American Journal of Public Health* 93, no. 12 (2003): 2067–2073.

Overdoses and substance abuse are a devastating part of my practice: Michael L. Barnett, Andrew R. Olenski, and Anupam B. Jena, "Opioid-Prescribing Patterns of Emergency Physicians and Risk of Long-Term Use," *New England Journal of Medicine* 376, no. 7 (2017): 663–673; Molly Moore Jeffery, W. Michael Hooten, Erik P. Hess, Ellen R. Meara, Joseph S. Ross, Henry J. Henk, Bjug Borgundvaag, Nilay D. Shah, and M. Fernanda Bellolio, "Opioid Prescribing for Opioid-Naive Patients in Emergency Departments and Other Settings: Characteristics of Prescriptions and Association with Long-Term Use," *Annals of Emergency Medicine* 71, no. 3 (2018): 326–336.

the tragic story of dental care inequality: Meredith Freed, Tricia Neuman, and Gretchen Jacobson, *Drilling Down on Dental Coverage and Costs for Medicare Beneficiaries* (Kaiser Family Foundation, 2019); Zoe Greenberg, "Our Teeth Are Making Us Sick," *New York Times*, Opinion Pages, May 23, 2017, https://kristof.blogs.nytimes.com/2017/05/23/our-teeth-are-making-us-sick/.

18   There's Dying, and Dying Now

An effective and meaningful process requires several elements to be in place: A. Fagerlin and C. E. Schneider, "Enough: The Failure of the Living Will," *Hastings Center Report* 34, no. 2 (March–April 2004): 30–42.

However, these documents may contain confusing or even contradictory instructions: T. A. Schmidt, D. Zive, E. K. Fromme, J. N. Cook, and S. W. Tolle, "Physician Orders for Life-Sustaining Treatment (Polst): Lessons Learned from Analysis of the Oregon Polst Registry," *Resuscitation* 85, no. 4 (2014): 480–485; B. Clemency, C. C. Cordes, H. A. Lindstrom, J. M. Basior, and D. P. Waldrop, "Decisions by Default: Incomplete and Contradictory

MOLST in Emergency Care," *Journal of American Medical Directors Association* 18, no. 1 (2017): 35–39.

But surrogates incorrectly predict patient preferences approximately one-third of the time: D. I. Shalowitz, E. Garrett-Mayer, and D. Wendler, "The Accuracy of Surrogate Decision Makers: A Systematic Review," *Archives of Internal Medicine* 166, no. 5 (2006): 493–497.

I'm dumbfounded that this [advanced care planning] information is often not readily available: Joshua R. Lakin, Eric Isaacs, Erin Sullivan, Heather A. Harris, Ryan D. McMahan, and Rebecca L. Sudore, "Emergency Physicians' Experience with Advance Care Planning Documentation in the Electronic Medical Record: Useful, Needed, and Elusive," *Journal of Palliative Medicine* 19, no. 6 (2016): 632–638; T. F. Platts-Mills, N. L. Richmond, E. M. LeFebvre, S. A. Mangipudi, A. G. Hollowell, D. Travers, K. Biese, L. C. Hanson, and A. E. Volandes, "Availability of Advance Care Planning Documentation for Older Emergency Department Patients: A Cross-Sectional Study," *Journal of Palliative Medicine* 20, no. 1 (2017): 74–78.

In a 1995 article, bioethicist Daniel Callahan wrote: Daniel Callahan, "Frustrated Mastery: The Cultural Context of Death in America," *Western Journal of Medicine* 163, no. 3 (1995): 226–230.

19   Holding On, Letting Go

Frankl wrote, "If there is a meaning in life at all . . .": Victor Frankl, *Man's Search for Meaning*, 4th ed. (Boston: Beacon Press, 2000).

"Do you think it's cowardice not to want to suffer?" Peter Richardson (dir.), *How to Die in Oregon*, 2011.

20   When Waiting Feels Immoral

Though studies cast an ugly shadow on notions of "objective" triage assessments by highlighting the influence of racial and gender bias: Lenny López, Andrew P. Wilper, Marina C. Cervantes, Joseph R. Betancourt, and Alexander R. Green, "Racial and Sex Differences in Emergency Department Triage Assessment and Test Ordering for Chest Pain, 1997–2006," *Academic Emergency Medicine* 17, no. 8 (2010): 801–808; Chet D. Schrader and

Lawrence M. Lewis, "Racial Disparity in Emergency Department Triage," *Journal of Emergency Medicine* 44, no. 2 (2013): 511–518.

our perception of waiting can feel as much as one-third longer: P. Jones, and Jen-Li Hwang, *Perceptions of Waiting Time in Different Service Queues* (Surrey Research Insight: University of Surrey, 2005).

In the ER, the perception of the wait contributes to patient dissatisfaction: D. A. Thompson, P. R. Yarnold, D. R. Williams, and S. L. Adams, "Effects of Actual Waiting Time, Perceived Waiting Time, Information Delivery, and Expressive Quality on Patient Satisfaction in the Emergency Department," *Annals of Emergency Medicine* 28, no. 6 (1996): 657–665.

In recent years, authors have coined the term "moral injury": Simon G. Talbot and Wendy Dean, "Physicians Aren't 'Burning Out.' They're Suffering from Moral Injury," *STAT*, July 26, 2018, https://www.statnews .com/2018/07/26/physicians-not-burning-out-they-are-suffering-moral -injury/.

21   Benefit Paradox

"One of our most difficult duties as human beings": Arthur Frank, *The Wounded Storyteller: Body, Illness, and Ethics* (Chicago: University of Chicago Press, 1997).

In his story "Gooseberries": Anton Chekhov, *Later Short Stories 1888–1903*, translated by Constance Garnett (New York: The Modern Library, 1999).

23   Big Incision

In her story "People Like That Are the Only People Here": Lorrie Moore, *Birds of America* (New York: Alfred A. Knopf, 1998).

24   To Err Is to Be a Physician

Most so-called experts are confident, even overconfident: Daniel Kahneman, *Thinking, Fast and Slow* (New York: Farrar, Straus and Giroux, 2011).

In one study, physicians were given easy and hard case vignettes: A. N. Meyer, V. L. Payne, D. W. Meeks, R. Rao, and H. Singh, "Physicians'

Diagnostic Accuracy, Confidence, and Resource Requests: A Vignette Study," *JAMA Internal Medicine* 173, no. 21(2013) 1952–1958.

When you're in the moment, being wrong feels a lot like being right: Kathryn Schulz, *Being Wrong: Adventures in the Margin of Error* (New York: Ecco Press, 2011).

Nancy Berlinger has described medical harm: Nancy Berlinger, *After Harm: Medical Error and the Ethics of Forgiveness* (Baltimore: The Johns Hopkins University Press, 2007).

In 1999, the Institute of Medicine (IOM) report: L. Kohn, J. Corrigan, and M. Donaldson, *To Err Is Human: Building a Safer Health System*, Committee on Quality of Health Care in America (Washington, DC: National Academies Press, 2000).

This overly broad definition muddies the relationship between poor outcomes and medical error: T. A. Brennan, "The Institute of Medicine Report on Medical Errors—Could It Do Harm?" *New England Journal of Medicine* 342, no. 15 (2000): 1123–1125.

Dr. Hardeep Singh and colleagues have developed a different paradigm: Hardeep Singh, "Editorial: Helping Health Care Organizations to Define Diagnostic Errors as Missed Opportunities in Diagnosis," *Joint Commission Journal of Quality and Patient Safety* 40, no. 3 (Mar 2014): 99–101.

28   Caring for the Caregiver

A large national survey revealed that one in five Americans serve as unpaid caregivers; close to 70 percent of caregivers are women; over 20 percent of caregivers in many states rate their own health as fair to poor: V. J. Edwards, E. D. Bouldin, C. A. Taylor, B. S. Olivari, and L. C. McGuire, "Characteristics and Health Status of Informal Unpaid Caregivers—44 States, District of Columbia, and Puerto Rico 2015–17," *Morbidity and Mortality Weekly Report* 69 (2020): 183–188; AARP and National Alliance for Caregiving, *Caregiving in the United States 2020* (Washington, DC: AARP, 2020).

A University of Michigan study showed that Medicare patients who are looked after by caregivers: Claire K. Ankuda, Donovan T. Maust,

Mohammed U. Kabeto, Ryan J. McCammon, Kenneth M. Langa, and Deborah A. Levine, "Association between Spousal Caregiver Well-Being and Care Recipient Healthcare Expenditures," *Journal of the American Geriatrics Society* 65, no. 10 (2017): 2220–2226.

dementia patients with caregivers suffering from symptoms of depression: Elan L. Guterman, I. Elaine Allen, S. Andrew Josephson, Jennifer J. Merrilees, Sarah Dulaney, Winston Chiong, Kirby Lee, et al., "Association between Caregiver Depression and Emergency Department Use among Patients with Dementia," *JAMA Neurology* 76, no. 10 (2019): 1166–1173.

The psychological distress and physical demands associated with caregiving are reflected in a disturbing range of biological responses:

slower wound healing: J. K. Kiecolt-Glaser, P. T. Marucha, A. M. Mercado, W. B. Malarkey, and R. Glaser, "Slowing of Wound Healing by Psychological Stress," *Lancet* 346, no. 8984 (1995): 1194–1196.

elevated blood pressure: Abby C. King, Roberta K Oka, and Deborah R. Young, "Ambulatory Blood Pressure and Heart Rate Responses to the Stress of Work and Caregiving in Older Women," *Journal of Gerontology* 49, no. 6 (1994): M239–M45.

impaired immune response: J. K. Kiecolt-Glaser, R. Glaser, S. Gravenstein, W. B. Malarkey, and J. Sheridan, "Chronic Stress Alters the Immune Response to Influenza Virus Vaccine in Older Adults," *Proceedings of the National Academy of Sciences of the United States of America* 93, no. 7 (1996): 3043–3047.

increase caregiver mortality: Richard Schulz and Scott R. Beach, "Caregiving as a Risk Factor for Mortality: The Caregiver Health Effects Study," *JAMA* 282, no. 23 (1999): 2215–2219.

Next Step in Care program produced by the United Hospital Fund: United Hospital Fund, "Next Step in Care: Family Caregivers and Health Care Professionals Working Together," https://www.nextstepincare.org/left_top _menu/Provider_Home/What_Do_I_Need; C. Levine, "Putting the Spotlight on Invisible Family Caregivers," *JAMA Internal Medicine* 176, no. 3 (2016): 380–381.

An estimated 14.7 million older adults receive assistance with daily activities from spouse and family caregivers: Jennifer L. Wolff, Brenda C Spillman, Vicki A. Freedman, and Judith D. Kasper, "A National Profile of Family and Unpaid Caregivers Who Assist Older Adults with Health Care Activities," *JAMA Internal Medicine* 176, no. 3 (2016): 372–379.

30   Dr. Douchebag

Tim O'Brien distinguishes "story" truth from "happening" truth: Tim O'Brien, *The Things They Carried* (New York: Penguin, 1990).

Emergency medicine was built on the "pillars of egalitarianism, social justice and compassion . . .": Brian Zink, *Anyone, Anything, Anytime: A History of Emergency Medicine*, 2nd. ed. (American College of Emergency Physicians, 2018); Brian Zink, "Social Justice, Egalitarianism, and the History of Emergency Medicine," *Virtual Mentor* 12, no. 6 (2010): 492–494.

"common courtesy, sincerity, and willingness to help": Gregory Luke Larkin, Kenneth Iserson, Zach Kassutto, Glenn Freas, Kathy Delaney, John Krimm, Terri Schmidt, et al., "Virtue in Emergency Medicine," *Academic Emergency Medicine* 16, no. 1 (2009): 51–55.

As Viktor Shklovsky pointed out in his famous 1917 essay: Viktor Shklovsky, *Theory of Prose*, translated by Benjamin Sher (Elmwood Park: Dalkey Archive Press, 1991).

what Charles Baxter has called "misfit details": Charles Baxter, "On Defamiliarization," in *Burning Down the House* (St. Paul, MN: Graywolf Press, 2008).

I also want to acknowledge my friends and colleagues Arno Kumagai and Delese Wear, who wrote beautifully about defamiliarization, the impact of automatic thinking on patient-centered care, and the importance of the arts and humanities in health professions education to "make strange— disturb and disrupt one's assumptions, perspectives and ways of acting so that one sees the self, others and the world anew": A. K. Kumagai and D. Wear, "'Making Strange': A Role for the Humanities in Medical Education," *Academic Medicine* 89, no. 7 (2014): 973–977.

31   In Defense of Cheaper Stethoscopes

The writer/critic Anatole Broyard said it best: "There is a paradox here at the heart of medicine": Anatole Broyard, *Intoxicated by My Illness* (New York: Fawcett Columbine, 1992).

Eric Topol . . . called the stethoscope nothing more than a pair of "rubber tubes": Lindsey Tanner, "Is the Stethoscope Dying? High-Tech Rivals Pose a Threat," *Washington Post*, November 12, 2019, https://www.washingtonpost.com/is-the-stethoscope-dying-high-tech-rivals-pose-a-threat/2019/11/08/4370ce84-f5c7-11e9-8cf0-4cc99f74d127_story.html.

32   The Appendix: Ancient Organ for the Modern Age

Researchers claim the appendix has evolved over thirty different times across multiple species: Midwestern University, "Appendix May Have Important Function, New Research Suggests," ScienceDaily, January 9, 2017, https://www.sciencedaily.com/releases/2017/01/170109162333.htm.

38   Can We Write a Better Story for Ourselves?

Today, physician productivity estimates suggest 20 to 30 percent of a physician's capacity: Christopher Kerns and Dave Willis, "The Problem with U.S. Health Care Isn't a Shortage of Doctors," *Harvard Business Review*, March 16, 2020, https://hbr.org/2020/03/the-problem-with-u-s-hea; Robert G. Hill, Lynn Marie Sears, and Scott W. Melanson, "4000 Clicks: A Productivity Analysis of Electronic Medical Records in a Community Hospital," *American Journal of Emergency Medicine* 31, no. 11 (2013): 1591–1594.

"We are what we pretend to be, so we must be careful about what we pretend to be": Kurt Vonnegut, *Mother Night* (New York: Dial Press, 1999).

In 1890, when Sir Henry Tate commissioned a painting from Luke Fildes: Heather Birchall, "The Doctor, Sir Luke Fildes, Exhibited 1891," accessed October 12, 2021, https://www.tate.org.uk/art/artworks/fildes-the-doctor-n01522.

39   Not an Ending

Chekhov said, "When I am finished with my characters, I like to return them to life," and Virginia Woolf quote on Chekhov: David Jauss, "Returning Characters to Life: Chekhov's Subversive Endings," *Writer's Chronicle* (March–April 2010).

There's provocative research that suggests a connection between readers' self-esteem and their comfort with certain endings: Silvia Knobloch-Westerwick and Caterina Keplinger, "Mystery Appeal: Effects of Uncertainty and Resolution on the Enjoyment of Mystery," *Media Psychology* 8, no. 3 (2006): 193–212.

The novelist E. L. Doctorow gave this now famous advice: George Plimpton, "E. L. Doctorow, the Art of Fiction No. 94," *Paris Review* no. 101 (Winter 1986).

40   Writing Stories of Medicine

The rewards of narrative writing, write journalists Mark Kramer and Wendy Call: "Introduction: Ethics," in *Telling True Stories*, edited by Mark Kramer and Wendy Call (New York: Plume, 2007).

"Narrative writers must strike a careful balance . . .": Isabel Wilkerson, "Playing Fair with Subjects," in *Telling True Stories*.

"was the thing which gained me entrance to those secret gardens of the self . . .": William Carlos Williams, *Autobiography* (New York: New Directions, 1951).

41   One Last Thing

six in ten healthcare workers said the stress from the pandemic harmed their mental health: William Wan, "Burned Out by the Pandemic, 3 in 10 Health-Care Workers Consider Leaving the Profession," *Washington Post*, April 22, 2021, https://www.washingtonpost.com/health/2021/04/22/health-workers-covid-quit/.

only 67 percent of people in the United States have received a dose of one of the COVID-19 vaccines: Centers for Disease Control and Prevention website, https://www.cdc.gov/coronavirus/2019-ncov/covid-data/covidview /index.html, accessed October 29, 2021.

The small piece was published in STAT on August 27, 2021: Jay Baruch, "It's Easy to Judge the Unvaccinated. As a Doctor, I See a Better Alternative," *STAT*, August 27, 2021, https://www.statnews.com/2021/08/27/its -easy-to-judge-the-unvaccinated-seek-a-better-alternative/.

a lack of trust in the vaccine development process, drawing on credibility problems with pharmaceutical companies: United States Department of Justice Website, "Justice Department Announces Largest Health Care Fraud Settlement in Its History," September 2, 2009, https://www.justice .gov/opa/pr/justice-department-announces-largest-health-care-fraud-settle ment-its-history.

that "place a patient or provider at risk of a poor outcome": J. L. Hick, D. Hanfling, M. Wynia, and E. Toner, "Crisis Standards of Care and COVID-19: What Did We Learn? How Do We Ensure Equity? What Should We Do?" *NAM Perspectives*, 2021. Discussion, National Academy of Medicine, Washington, DC, https://doi.org/10.31478/202108e.

Some overwhelmed hospitals transferred patients to open beds in ICUs: Heather Hollingsworth and Jim Saltre, "With No Beds, Hospitals Ship Patients to Far-Off Cities," Associated Press, August 18, 2021, https:// apnews.com/article/health-coronavirus-pandemic-0ba6aa292483a89d52 ab44b5f5434815.

To persuade people, to get them to think, you must first get them to understand: Robert McKee and Bronwyn Fryer, "Storytelling That Moves People," *Harvard Business Review* 81, no. 6 (2003): 51–55.

Index